OWEN HUNTER

Hidradenitis Suppurativa

Your Comprehensive Blueprint for Diagnosis and Treatment

Contents

INTRODUCTION

Hidradenitis Suppurativa: Reclaiming Your Life from a Debilitating Skin Condition

Imagine living with a chronic, painful skin condition that not only affects your physical well-being but also takes a toll on your mental health, social relationships, and overall quality of life. This is the reality for the millions of individuals worldwide who suffer from Hidradenitis Suppurativa (HS), a complex and often misunderstood inflammatory skin disease.

Hidradenitis Suppurativa is a lifelong, recurrent condition characterized by the development of painful, pus-filled lesions, abscesses, and sinus tracts in the body's apocrine sweat gland-bearing areas, such as the armpits, groin, and buttocks. While the exact causes of HS are not fully understood, it is believed to involve a combination of genetic, hormonal, and environmental factors that lead to chronic inflammation and the obstruction of hair follicles.

For those living with HS, the physical symptoms can be debilitating, with painful flare-ups that can significantly impact daily activities and quality of life. The disease not only causes significant physical discomfort but also often leads to social isolation, low self-esteem, and mental health challenges such as depression and anxiety.

Despite the significant burden HS places on those affected, it remains a widely misunderstood and underdiagnosed condition. Many individuals struggle for years, often facing misdiagnosis or inadequate treatment options, before finally receiving the appropriate care and support they need.

This book, "Hidradenitis Suppurativa: Reclaiming Your Life from a Debilitating Skin Condition," is designed to be a comprehensive guide that empowers individuals living with HS to take control of their health and reclaim their lives. Through this in-depth exploration of the condition, we will delve into the latest research, treatment options, and strategies for managing the physical and emotional aspects of this complex disease.

The journey towards better understanding and managing Hidradenitis Suppurativa is not an easy one, but it is a journey worth taking. By equipping readers with the knowledge, tools, and resources they need, this book aims to provide a roadmap for those living with HS to navigate the challenges they face and ultimately achieve a better quality of life.

Chapter by chapter, we will explore the various facets of Hidradenitis Suppurativa, from the underlying causes and symptoms to the latest advancements in diagnosis and treatment. We will also delve into the impact of HS on mental health, the importance of a multidisciplinary approach to care, and strategies for managing flare-ups and long-term complications.

Through personal stories, expert insights, and evidence-based information, this book will serve as a comprehensive resource for individuals with Hidradenitis Suppurativa, their loved ones, and healthcare professionals seeking to provide the most effective care.

Whether you have recently been diagnosed with HS or have been living with the condition for years, this book is designed to be your trusted companion on the path to reclaiming your life and achieving the best possible outcomes.

Understanding Hidradenitis Suppurativa: A Complex and Debilitating Skin

Condition

Hidradenitis Suppurativa, also known as acne inversa, is a chronic, inflammatory skin condition that affects an estimated 1-4% of the global population. While the exact prevalence is difficult to determine due to underdiagnosis and lack of awareness, it is clear that HS is a significant public health concern that deserves greater attention and understanding.

The hallmark symptoms of Hidradenitis Suppurativa are the development of painful, recurrent lesions, abscesses, and sinus tracts in the body's apocrine sweat gland-bearing areas, such as the armpits, groin, and buttocks. These lesions often begin as small, painful bumps or boils that can progress to larger, interconnected abscesses and draining fistulas. The chronic nature of the condition means that individuals with HS often experience a cycle of flare-ups and remissions, with periods of relative calm punctuated by sudden, debilitating outbreaks.

The physical symptoms of Hidradenitis Suppurativa can be truly debilitating, causing significant pain, discomfort, and impairment of daily activities. The lesions and abscesses can be so painful that even the most mundane tasks, such as getting dressed or using the bathroom, become agonizing ordeals. Additionally, the chronic nature of the condition and the unsightly appearance of the lesions can lead to social isolation, embarrassment, and a profound impact on overall quality of life.

Beyond the physical manifestations, Hidradenitis Suppurativa also takes a significant toll on the mental and emotional well-being of those affected. The constant pain, disfigurement, and social stigma associated with the condition can lead to depression, anxiety, and a profound sense of hopelessness. Many individuals with HS report feeling misunderstood, stigmatized, and unsupported by healthcare providers and their own social circles.

Despite the significant burden Hidradenitis Suppurativa places on those affected, the condition remains widely misunderstood and underdiagnosed. Many individuals struggle for years, often facing multiple misdiagnoses or inadequate treatment options, before finally receiving the appropriate care and support they need.

This lack of awareness and understanding surrounding HS is, in part, due to the complex and multifaceted nature of the condition. The underlying causes of Hidradenitis Suppurativa are not yet fully understood, with a combination of genetic, hormonal, and environmental factors believed to play a role in the development and progression of the disease.

Additionally, the heterogeneous presentation of HS, with varying degrees of severity and symptom patterns, can make it challenging for healthcare providers to recognize and diagnose the condition, further contributing to the underdiagnosis and delayed treatment experienced by many patients.

It is against this backdrop that this book, "Hidradenitis Suppurativa: Reclaiming Your Life from a Debilitating Skin Condition," has been written. By providing a comprehensive guide to understanding, managing, and living with this complex and often misunderstood condition, we aim to empower individuals with Hidradenitis Suppurativa to take control of their health and reclaim their lives.

Through a deep dive into the latest research, treatment options, and strategies for managing the physical and emotional aspects of HS, this book will serve as a valuable resource for those living with the condition, as well as their loved ones and healthcare providers.

Our goal is to shed light on the often-overlooked challenges faced by individuals with Hidradenitis Suppurativa, while also offering hope and practical solutions for navigating the journey towards better health and quality of life.

By the end of this book, readers will have a thorough understanding of Hidradenitis Suppurativa, from its underlying causes to the most cutting-edge treatment approaches. More importantly, they will be equipped with the knowledge, tools, and resources they need to take an active role in managing their condition and reclaiming their lives from the debilitating effects of this complex skin disease.

CHAPTER 1

Understanding Hidradenitis Suppurativa

Unveiling the Mysteries of a Complex Skin Condition

Hidradenitis Suppurativa (HS) is a chronic, recurrent, and often debilitating skin condition that can have a profound impact on the lives of those affected. Also known as acne inversa, HS is characterized by the development of painful, inflamed lesions, abscesses, and sinus tracts in the body's apocrine sweat gland-bearing areas, such as the armpits, groin, and buttocks.

To truly understand this complex condition, we must first delve into the definition, prevalence, and underlying causes of Hidradenitis Suppurativa. By exploring these fundamental aspects, we can begin to unravel the mysteries surrounding this often-misunderstood skin disease and set the stage for a comprehensive exploration of its impact, diagnosis, and management.

Defining Hidradenitis Suppurativa

Hidradenitis Suppurativa is a chronic, inflammatory skin condition that is characterized by the development of recurrent, painful lesions and abscesses in the body's apocrine sweat gland-bearing areas. These lesions typically begin as small, painful bumps or boils that can progress to larger, interconnected abscesses and draining fistulas.

The word "hidradenitis" refers to the inflammation of the sweat glands, while "suppurativa" describes the pus-filled nature of the lesions. This combination of chronic inflammation and recurrent, purulent lesions is the hallmark of Hidradenitis Suppurativa, setting it apart from other skin conditions.

One of the unique aspects of HS is its predilection for specific anatomical locations, namely the apocrine sweat gland-bearing areas of the body. These include the armpits, groin, buttocks, and sometimes the breasts, genitals, and other intertriginous (skin-to-skin) areas. The concentration of apocrine sweat glands in these regions is believed to play a crucial role in the development and progression of the disease.

It is important to note that Hidradenitis Suppurativa is a chronic, recurrent condition, meaning that individuals with HS often experience a cycle of flare-ups and remissions throughout their lives. The severity and frequency of these flare-ups can vary greatly, with some individuals experiencing milder, less frequent episodes and others facing more severe, debilitating outbreaks.

Prevalence and Demographic Factors

Hidradenitis Suppurativa is a relatively common skin condition, affecting an estimated 1-4% of the global population. However, the true prevalence of HS is difficult to determine, as the condition is often underdiagnosed or misdiagnosed, leading to a significant number of undiagnosed cases.

While HS can affect individuals of any age, gender, or ethnicity, certain demographic factors have been associated with an increased risk of developing the condition. For instance, HS is more commonly diagnosed in women than in men, with a female-to-male ratio ranging from 3:1 to 5:1.

The onset of Hidradenitis Suppurativa typically occurs during the late teens to early 40s, with the peak incidence observed between the ages of 20 and 30. However, it is important to note that HS can also develop in children and adolescents, as well as in older adults.

Certain ethnic and geographic variations in the prevalence of Hidradenitis Suppurativa have also been observed. Studies have suggested that HS may be more common in populations of African descent, as well as in certain regions of the world, such as Northern Europe and the Middle East.

Underlying Causes and Pathophysiology

The exact causes of Hidradenitis Suppurativa are not yet fully understood, but it is believed to involve a complex interplay of genetic, hormonal, and environmental factors that lead to chronic inflammation and the obstruction of hair follicles.

Genetic Factors
Numerous studies have indicated that genetic predisposition plays a significant role in the development of Hidradenitis Suppurativa. Individuals with a family history of HS are at a higher risk of developing the condition, suggesting a strong genetic component.

Several genetic mutations have been associated with Hidradenitis Suppurativa, including those involving the gamma-secretase complex, which is involved in the regulation of cellular signaling and inflammation. Additionally, variants in genes related to the immune system and skin barrier function have also been linked to an increased risk of HS.

It is important to note that the inheritance pattern of Hidradenitis Suppurativa is not entirely clear, and the condition is not considered a simple, single-gene disorder. Rather, it is believed to involve a complex interplay of multiple genetic factors, each contributing to the overall risk and severity of the disease.

Hormonal Factors

Hormonal influences are also believed to play a significant role in the development and progression of Hidradenitis Suppurativa. The higher incidence of HS in women, particularly during the reproductive years, suggests that hormonal factors, such as fluctuations in estrogen, testosterone, and other sex hormones, may contribute to the condition.

The link between hormones and Hidradenitis Suppurativa is further supported by the observation that HS often improves during pregnancy and worsens during the postpartum period. Additionally, certain hormonal contraceptives and medications that affect hormone levels have been shown to influence the course of the disease.

Researchers are actively investigating the specific mechanisms by which hormonal factors contribute to the development and progression of Hidradenitis Suppurativa, with the aim of developing more targeted, hormone-based treatment approaches.

Environmental and Lifestyle Factors

In addition to genetic and hormonal influences, environmental and lifestyle factors have also been implicated in the development of Hidradenitis Suppurativa. Factors such as obesity, smoking, and stress have been consistently associated with an increased risk and severity of the condition.

Obesity, in particular, is a well-established risk factor for Hidradenitis Suppurativa. The excess adipose tissue in obese individuals is believed to contribute to chronic inflammation, which can exacerbate the symptoms of HS. Additionally, the friction and irritation caused by skin-to-skin contact in areas with increased adiposity may further aggravate the condition.

Smoking, on the other hand, is thought to impact the immune system and skin barrier function, potentially increasing the risk of developing Hidradenitis Suppurativa and contributing to its severity. The relationship between stress and HS is less well-understood, but it is believed that chronic stress can trigger or worsen flare-ups by altering the body's inflammatory response.

Pathophysiology of Hidradenitis Suppurativa
   The underlying pathophysiology of Hidradenitis Suppurativa is complex and not yet fully elucidated, but it is believed to involve a combination of follicular occlusion, inflammation, and immune system dysregulation.

One of the key pathogenic mechanisms in HS is the obstruction of the hair follicles, particularly in the apocrine sweat gland-bearing areas. This follicular occlusion is thought to lead to the development of keratin plugs, which can trap bacteria and trigger an inflammatory response.

The inflammatory process in Hidradenitis Suppurativa is characterized by the infiltration of immune cells, such as neutrophils and lymphocytes, into the affected skin. This inflammatory cascade leads to the formation of painful, pus-filled lesions and abscesses, which can further contribute to the obstruction and destruction of the hair follicles and surrounding tissue.

Underlying this inflammatory response is believed to be an imbalance or dysregulation of the immune system, which may be influenced by genetic, hormonal, and environmental factors. Researchers have identified various inflammatory mediators, such as cytokines and chemokines, that play a crucial role in the pathogenesis of HS.

The chronic, recurrent nature of Hidradenitis Suppurativa is thought to be driven by the persistent inflammation and the formation of sinus tracts, which can connect the affected areas and lead to the development of new lesions. This cycle of inflammation, tissue damage, and new lesion formation is a hallmark of the disease and contributes to the significant burden experienced by individuals with HS.

Understanding the underlying causes and pathophysiology of Hidradenitis

Suppurativa is essential for the development of effective treatment strategies and the implementation of preventive measures. By unraveling the complex interplay of genetic, hormonal, and environmental factors that contribute to the condition, researchers and healthcare providers can work towards a more personalized and holistic approach to managing this debilitating skin disease.

The Impact of Hidradenitis Suppurativa

Hidradenitis Suppurativa is a condition that can have a profound and far-reaching impact on the lives of those affected. Beyond the physical symptoms, HS can also take a significant toll on an individual's emotional, social, and overall quality of life.

Physical Burden

The primary physical manifestations of Hidradenitis Suppurativa, such as the development of painful, recurrent lesions and abscesses, can be truly debilitating. The chronic nature of the condition means that individuals with HS often experience a cycle of flare-ups and remissions, with periods of relative calm punctuated by sudden, debilitating outbreaks.

These painful lesions and abscesses can significantly impair an individual's ability to perform even the most basic daily tasks, such as getting dressed, using the bathroom, or engaging in physical activity. The discomfort and limitations imposed by the physical symptoms of HS can lead to a profound impact on an individual's overall quality of life and well-being.

Emotional and Psychological Impact

In addition to the physical burden, Hidradenitis Suppurativa can also have a significant impact on an individual's emotional and psychological well-being. The constant pain, disfigurement, and social stigma associated with the condition can lead to a range of mental health challenges, such as depression, anxiety, and feelings of low self-esteem.

Many individuals with HS report feeling misunderstood, stigmatized, and unsupported by healthcare providers and their own social circles. The visible nature of the lesions and the sometimes-unpleasant odor associated with the condition can contribute to feelings of embarrassment, shame, and social isolation.

The emotional toll of Hidradenitis Suppurativa can be particularly pronounced, as the condition often affects individuals during their formative years, when social connections and self-image are of great importance. The impact of HS on an individual's mental health and overall well-being cannot be overstated, and addressing these emotional challenges is a critical component of comprehensive care for those living with the condition.

Social and Occupational Implications

The physical and emotional burdens of Hidradenitis Suppurativa can also have significant social and occupational implications for those affected. The pain, discomfort, and disfigurement associated with the condition can make it challenging for individuals to participate in social activities, maintain employment, or pursue educational or career goals.

The recurrent nature of HS flare-ups can also lead to frequent absences from work or school, further exacerbating the social and occupational challenges faced by those living with the condition. Additionally, the stigma and misunderstanding surrounding HS can make it difficult for individuals to openly discuss their condition with employers, colleagues, or peers, leading to feelings of isolation and marginalization.

The impact of Hidradenitis Suppurativa on an individual's social and occupational functioning can have far-reaching consequences, affecting not only their immediate quality of life but also their long-term personal and professional development.

Recognizing and addressing the multifaceted impact of HS is essential for providing comprehensive, holistic care to those affected by this debilitating skin condition. By understanding the physical, emotional, and social challenges faced by individuals with Hidradenitis Suppurativa, healthcare providers, policymakers, and society as a whole can work to develop more effective strategies for supporting and empowering those living with this complex and often misunderstood disease.

Conclusion

Hidradenitis Suppurativa is a chronic, inflammatory skin condition that can have a profound and wide-ranging impact on the lives of those affected. From the physical symptoms of painful lesions and abscesses to the emotional and social challenges posed by the condition, HS can significantly impair an individual's overall quality of life.

By delving into the definition, prevalence, and underlying causes of Hidradenitis Suppurativa, we have laid the groundwork for a deeper understanding of this complex and often misunderstood skin disease. The genetic, hormonal, and environmental factors that contribute to the development and progression of HS highlight the multifaceted nature of the condition and the need for a comprehensive, personalized approach to management.

Moreover, exploring the substantial impact of Hidradenitis Suppurativa on physical, emotional, and social well-being underscores the importance of addressing the holistic needs of individuals living with this debilitating condition. As we move forward in our exploration of HS, this foundational knowledge will serve as a crucial guide for navigating the complexities of diagnosis, treatment, and long-term management.

With a deeper understanding of Hidradenitis Suppurativa, we are now poised to embark on a journey towards empowering those affected by this condition and supporting them in their quest to reclaim their lives. By continuing to unravel the mysteries of HS and advocating for greater awareness and better care, we can work towards a future where individuals with Hidradenitis Suppurativa are no longer burdened by the physical, emotional, and social challenges of this complex skin disease.

CHAPTER 2

S ymptoms and Stages of Hidradenitis Suppurativa

Navigating the Complexities of a Chronic, Recurrent Skin Condition

Hidradenitis Suppurativa (HS) is a complex and often misunderstood skin condition that presents with a wide range of symptoms and follows a distinct progression through various stages. Understanding the hallmark symptoms and the stages of HS is crucial for accurate diagnosis, effective management, and empowering individuals living with this chronic, recurrent disease.

In this chapter, we will delve into the common symptoms associated with Hidradenitis Suppurativa, exploring how they manifest and evolve over time. We will then examine the distinct stages of the condition, providing a comprehensive overview of the disease's progression and the unique characteristics of each stage. By enhancing our understanding of the clinical presentation of HS, we can better equip individuals affected by the condition to recognize, manage, and advocate for their unique healthcare needs.

Common Symptoms of Hidradenitis Suppurativa

The primary symptoms of Hidradenitis Suppurativa are centered around the development of painful, recurrent lesions, abscesses, and sinus tracts in the body's apocrine sweat gland-bearing areas. These include the armpits, groin, buttocks, and sometimes the breasts, genitals, and other intertriginous (skin-to-skin) regions.

Painful Lesions and Abscesses

The hallmark symptom of Hidradenitis Suppurativa is the development of painful, inflamed lesions and abscesses. These often begin as small, painful bumps or boils that can progress to larger, interconnected abscesses and draining fistulas (sinus tracts).

The pain associated with these lesions and abscesses can be severe, often described as a burning, throbbing, or stabbing sensation. The intensity of the pain can significantly impair an individual's ability to perform even the most basic daily activities, such as getting dressed, using the bathroom, or engaging in physical exercise.

In addition to the physical discomfort, the appearance of these lesions and abscesses can also be distressing, leading to feelings of embarrassment, self-consciousness, and social isolation.

Recurrent Nature and Flare-ups

A key characteristic of Hidradenitis Suppurativa is its chronic, recurrent nature. Individuals with HS often experience a cycle of flare-ups and remissions, with periods of relative calm punctuated by sudden, debilitating outbreaks of the condition.

The frequency and severity of these flare-ups can vary greatly among individuals, with some experiencing milder, less frequent episodes and others facing more severe, disabling outbreaks. The unpredictable nature of these flare-ups can make it challenging for individuals with HS to plan and engage in daily activities, further contributing to the burden of the condition.

Sinus Tract Formation

As Hidradenitis Suppurativa progresses, the development of sinus tracts, or fistulas, becomes a common occurrence. These interconnected, draining tunnels can form between the affected skin areas, leading to the formation of larger, more complex lesions and abscesses.

The presence of sinus tracts can further exacerbate the pain and discomfort associated with HS, as well as increase the risk of infection and the potential for scarring and disfigurement. The chronic, persistent nature of these sinus tracts is a hallmark of advanced Hidradenitis Suppurativa and can significantly impact an individual's quality of life.

Odor and Drainage

Another common symptom associated with Hidradenitis Suppurativa is the presence of drainage and an unpleasant odor from the affected areas. As the lesions and abscesses rupture or drain, they can release pus, blood, and other fluids, which can lead to a distinctive, often foul-smelling odor.

This symptom can be particularly distressing for individuals with HS, as it can contribute to feelings of self-consciousness, social discomfort, and further isolation. The drainage and odor associated with HS can also increase the risk of secondary infections and complicate the management of the condition.

Skin Changes and Scarring

Over time, the chronic inflammation and recurrent lesions of Hidradenitis Suppurativa can lead to significant changes in the affected skin. These changes may include thickening, discoloration, and the development of hypertrophic or keloid scarring.

The scarring and skin changes associated with HS can be disfiguring and further contribute to the emotional and social challenges faced by individuals living with the condition. These visible manifestations of the disease can exacerbate feelings of self-consciousness, low self-esteem, and social isolation.

Recognizing and understanding the diverse array of symptoms associated with Hidradenitis Suppurativa is crucial for early detection, accurate diagnosis, and the implementation of appropriate management strategies. By empowering individuals with HS to identify and articulate their symptoms, we can help them navigate the complexities of this chronic, recurrent skin condition and advocate for the care and support they need.

Stages of Hidradenitis Suppurativa

Hidradenitis Suppurativa is a chronic, progressive condition that typically follows a distinct pattern of disease progression, characterized by several well-defined stages. Understanding these stages is essential for accurately diagnosing HS, monitoring the condition's evolution, and tailoring treatment approaches to the specific needs of each individual.

The Hurley Staging System

The Hurley Staging System is the most widely recognized and utilized tool for classifying the stages of Hidradenitis Suppurativa. This system categorizes the condition into three distinct stages based on the severity of the clinical presentation and the extent of the disease.

Stage I: Mild

The first stage of Hidradenitis Suppurativa, known as Stage I or Mild, is characterized by the presence of isolated, single or multiple, abscess formations without sinus tracts or scarring.

In this early stage, individuals may experience the development of painful, inflamed lesions or boils, typically in a single, localized area, such as the armpit or groin. These lesions may drain or resolve spontaneously, but they do not progress to the formation of interconnected abscesses or sinus tracts.

The skin changes in Stage I HS are relatively limited, and the condition is generally considered the mildest form of the disease. However, even at this early stage, the recurrent nature of the condition and the associated pain can have a significant impact on an individual's quality of life.

Stage II: Moderate

As Hidradenitis Suppurativa progresses, it can advance to Stage II, or the Moderate stage. In this stage, individuals typically present with recurrent abscesses, with widely separated, single or multiple, well-defined lesions, and the formation of sinus tracts and scarring.

The key distinguishing feature of Stage II HS is the presence of interconnected abscesses and sinus tracts, which can lead to the development of larger, more complex lesions. These sinus tracts may connect the affected areas, creating a network of tunnels and contributing to the chronic, recurrent nature of the condition.

The skin changes in Stage II HS are more pronounced, with the development of scarring and the potential for increased disfigurement. The severity of the symptoms, including pain, drainage, and odor, can also be more pronounced in this stage of the disease.

Stage III: Severe

In the most advanced stage of Hidradenitis Suppurativa, known as Stage III or Severe, individuals present with diffuse or near-diffuse involvement of the affected areas, characterized by multiple interconnected sinus tracts and abscesses, as well as substantial scarring.

The hallmark of Stage III HS is the extensive involvement and interconnectedness of the affected areas, which can lead to a significant impact on an individual's physical, emotional, and social well-being. The pain, drainage, and disfigurement associated with this stage of the condition can be particularly debilitating, often requiring specialized, multidisciplinary care.

In addition to the physical symptoms, individuals with Stage III HS may also face an increased risk of complications, such as the development of fistulas (abnormal connections between organs or tissues) and the potential for malignant transformations, further emphasizing the need for comprehensive, proactive management.

It is important to note that the progression of Hidradenitis Suppurativa is not linear, and individuals may experience fluctuations between stages, with periods of relative calm followed by sudden, severe flare-ups. The Hurley Staging System provides a framework for understanding the evolution of the condition, but it is not always a perfect predictor of an individual's disease course or response to treatment.

By familiarizing ourselves with the distinct stages of Hidradenitis Suppurativa and the associated clinical presentations, we can better equip individuals living with HS to recognize the progression of their condition, advocate for timely and appropriate care, and collaborate with healthcare providers to develop personalized management strategies.

The Importance of Accurate Diagnosis

Accurately diagnosing Hidradenitis Suppurativa is crucial for ensuring appropriate treatment, monitoring disease progression, and empowering individuals to manage their condition effectively. However, the diagnosis of HS can be challenging, as the condition can often be misdiagnosed or overlooked due to a lack of awareness and understanding among healthcare providers.

One of the primary challenges in diagnosing Hidradenitis Suppurativa is the variability in its clinical presentation. The symptoms of HS can mimic those of other skin conditions, such as boils, folliculitis, or even inflammatory bowel disease, leading to potential misdiagnosis or delayed diagnosis.

Moreover, the chronic, recurrent nature of HS, with periods of flare-ups and remissions, can further complicate the diagnostic process, as individuals may seek medical attention only during acute episodes, rather than during periods of relative calm.

To overcome these challenges, healthcare providers must be equipped with a thorough understanding of the hallmark symptoms and stages of Hidradenitis Suppurativa, as well as a willingness to consider HS as a potential diagnosis, particularly in individuals presenting with recurrent, painful lesions in the apocrine sweat gland-bearing areas.

Establishing a diagnosis of Hidradenitis Suppurativa typically involves a comprehensive clinical evaluation, including a detailed medical history, physical examination, and, in some cases, diagnostic imaging or laboratory testing. The presence of the characteristic lesions, abscesses, and sinus tracts, as well as the involvement of the typical anatomical locations, are key diagnostic criteria for HS.

By promoting awareness and education about the diverse presentation of Hidradenitis Suppurativa, we can empower healthcare providers to recognize and accurately diagnose this condition, ultimately leading to more timely and appropriate care for individuals living with HS.

Conclusion

Hidradenitis Suppurativa is a complex, chronic skin condition that presents with a wide array of symptoms and follows a distinct pattern of disease progression. Understanding the hallmark symptoms, such as painful lesions, recurrent flare-ups, sinus tract formation, and skin changes, is crucial for recognizing and managing this condition effectively.

The Hurley Staging System provides a comprehensive framework for categorizing the stages of Hidradenitis Suppurativa, from the mild, early-stage presentations to the severe, advanced forms of the disease. By familiarizing ourselves with these stages and their associated clinical characteristics, we can better equip individuals living with HS to recognize the evolution of their condition, advocate for appropriate care, and collaborate with healthcare providers to develop personalized management strategies.

Accurate diagnosis is a fundamental step in the management of Hidradenitis Suppurativa, as it allows for the implementation of targeted, evidence-based treatment approaches. However, the variability in the clinical presentation of HS and the potential for misdiagnosis highlight the importance of healthcare provider education and the empowerment of individuals affected by this condition to advocate for timely and appropriate care.

By enhancing our understanding of the symptoms and stages of Hidradenitis Suppurativa, we can better support those living with this chronic, recurrent skin condition, enabling them to navigate the complexities of their disease and reclaim their quality of life. This knowledge will serve as a crucial foundation as we explore the multifaceted aspects of HS management in the chapters that follow.

CHAPTER 3

R isk Factors and Triggers for Hidradenitis Suppurativa

Unraveling the Complexities of a Multifactorial Skin Condition

Hidradenitis Suppurativa (HS) is a complex, chronic skin condition that is influenced by a variety of risk factors and triggers. Understanding these contributing elements is crucial for individuals living with HS, as it allows them to better manage their condition, minimize flare-ups, and take proactive steps towards improving their overall health and well-being.

In this chapter, we will delve into the various risk factors and triggers associated with Hidradenitis Suppurativa, exploring the genetic, hormonal, and environmental factors that can contribute to the development and progression of this debilitating skin condition. By examining these key elements, we can empower individuals with HS to recognize the potential influencers of their disease, implement targeted prevention strategies, and collaborate with healthcare providers to develop personalized management plans.

Genetic Predisposition

One of the well-established risk factors for Hidradenitis Suppurativa is a genetic predisposition. Numerous studies have indicated that individuals with a family history of HS are at a significantly higher risk of developing the condition, suggesting a strong genetic component.

The inheritance pattern of Hidradenitis Suppurativa is not straightforward, as it is not considered a simple, single-gene disorder. Rather, it is believed to involve a complex interplay of multiple genetic factors, each contributing to the overall risk and severity of the disease.

Several specific genetic mutations and variants have been associated with an increased susceptibility to Hidradenitis Suppurativa. These include:

1. Gamma-Secretase Complex: Mutations in genes involved in the gamma-secretase complex, a crucial regulator of cellular signaling and inflammation, have been linked to the development of HS.

2. Immune System Genes: Variations in genes related to immune system function, such as those involved in the regulation of cytokines and chemokines, have been implicated in the pathogenesis of Hidradenitis Suppurativa.

3. Skin Barrier Genes: Genetic alterations affecting the skin barrier function, including genes responsible for the production of structural proteins and lipids, have also been associated with an increased risk of HS.

The genetic underpinnings of Hidradenitis Suppurativa are an active area of research, and ongoing studies continue to uncover new genetic factors that may contribute to the condition. By identifying the specific genetic markers associated with HS, researchers and healthcare providers can work towards developing more targeted, personalized approaches to prevention and treatment.

It is important to note that the presence of a genetic predisposition does not necessarily guarantee the development of Hidradenitis Suppurativa. The interaction between genetic factors and environmental or hormonal influences can play a significant role in the actual manifestation of the condition. However, individuals with a family history of HS should be aware of their increased risk and proactively engage with healthcare providers to monitor for early signs of the condition and implement appropriate management strategies.

Hormonal Factors

Hormonal influences are another well-recognized risk factor for the development and progression of Hidradenitis Suppurativa. The higher prevalence of HS in women, particularly during the reproductive years, suggests that fluctuations in sex hormones, such as estrogen, testosterone, and their metabolites, may contribute to the onset and exacerbation of the condition.

The link between hormones and Hidradenitis Suppurativa is further supported by the observation that the condition often improves during pregnancy and worsens during the postpartum period. Additionally, certain hormonal contraceptives and medications that affect hormone levels have been shown to influence the course of the disease.

The precise mechanisms by which hormonal factors contribute to the development and progression of Hidradenitis Suppurativa are not yet fully understood, but researchers have proposed several potential pathways:

1. Hormonal Regulation of Sebum Production: Sex hormones, such as testosterone and its metabolites, can influence the production of sebum (oil) in the skin. Increased sebum production may contribute to the obstruction of hair follicles, a key pathogenic mechanism in HS.

2. Hormonal Modulation of Inflammation: Hormones, particularly estrogen and testosterone, can impact the immune system and the inflammatory response, potentially exacerbating the chronic inflammation associated with Hidradenitis Suppurativa.

3. Hormonal Effects on Skin Structure and Function: Hormonal fluctuations can affect the structure and function of the skin, including the activity of the apocrine sweat glands, which are central to the development of HS lesions.

The recognition of the hormonal component in Hidradenitis Suppurativa has led to the exploration of targeted, hormone-based treatment approaches, such as the use of anti-androgen therapies, oral contraceptives, and hormone-modulating medications. However, the individual response to these interventions can vary, highlighting the need for a personalized approach to managing the hormonal aspects of HS.

Individuals with Hidradenitis Suppurativa, particularly women, should be aware of the potential role of hormonal factors in their condition and work closely with their healthcare providers to monitor and manage any hormonal imbalances or fluctuations that may contribute to their disease progression.

Environmental and Lifestyle Factors

In addition to genetic and hormonal influences, environmental and lifestyle factors have also been identified as significant risk factors for the development and exacerbation of Hidradenitis Suppurativa.

Obesity

Obesity is a well-established risk factor for Hidradenitis Suppurativa. Numerous studies have consistently demonstrated a strong association between excess body weight and an increased risk of developing HS, as well as a higher likelihood of experiencing more severe disease progression.

The underlying mechanisms by which obesity contributes to Hidradenitis Suppurativa are multifaceted. The excess adipose tissue in obese individuals is believed to contribute to chronic low-grade inflammation, which can exacerbate the inflammatory processes underlying HS. Additionally, the increased friction and irritation caused by skin-to-skin contact in areas with increased adiposity may further aggravate the condition.

Smoking

Smoking is another significant risk factor for Hidradenitis Suppurativa. Numerous studies have consistently demonstrated that individuals who smoke are at a higher risk of developing HS and are more likely to experience more severe disease progression.

The exact mechanisms by which smoking influences the development and course of Hidradenitis Suppurativa are not fully understood, but several potential pathways have been proposed:

1. Immune System Dysregulation: Tobacco smoke exposure can alter the function of the immune system, potentially contributing to the chronic inflammation and immune dysregulation observed in HS.

2. Impaired Skin Barrier Function: Smoking can have detrimental effects on the skin barrier, potentially increasing the risk of follicular occlusion and the development of HS lesions.

3. Vascular Damage: Smoking can cause vascular damage and impair blood flow, which may compromise the skin's ability to heal and regenerate, further exacerbating the condition.

Stress

While the relationship between stress and Hidradenitis Suppurativa is less well-established, there is growing evidence suggesting that chronic stress may be a contributing factor to the development and exacerbation of the condition.

Stress can trigger or worsen HS flare-ups by altering the body's inflammatory response and potentially affecting the immune system. The physiological and psychological effects of chronic stress can lead to increased inflammation, hormonal imbalances, and disruptions in the skin's barrier function, all of which may contribute to the pathogenesis of Hidradenitis Suppurativa.

It is important to note that the impact of stress on HS is complex and may vary among individuals. Some may experience a direct correlation between stress levels and disease flare-ups, while others may not observe a clear association. Nonetheless, addressing and managing stress, through techniques such as mindfulness, relaxation practices, and mental health support, may be a valuable component of a comprehensive HS management plan.

Other Factors

In addition to obesity, smoking, and stress, other environmental and lifestyle factors have also been linked to an increased risk of Hidradenitis Suppurativa, including:

- Poor hygiene: Inadequate hygiene and skin care practices may contribute to the development of HS by promoting the accumulation of bacteria and the obstruction of hair follicles.

- Mechanical irritation: Repetitive friction or trauma to the skin, such as from tight clothing or shaving, may exacerbate the condition.

- Certain medications: Some medications, such as lithium and certain biologics, have been associated with an increased risk of developing HS.

- Climate and geography: There may be regional or geographic variations in the prevalence of Hidradenitis Suppurativa, potentially due to environmental factors or lifestyle differences.

Understanding the multifaceted risk factors and triggers for Hidradenitis Suppurativa is crucial for empowering individuals living with the condition to take an active role in managing their disease. By recognizing the genetic, hormonal, and environmental factors that may contribute to their HS, individuals can work with their healthcare providers to implement targeted prevention strategies, minimize flare-ups, and optimize their overall health and well-being.

Implications for Prevention and Management

The recognition of the various risk factors and triggers associated with Hidradenitis Suppurativa has significant implications for the prevention and management of this chronic, debilitating skin condition.

Prevention Strategies

By identifying the key risk factors for Hidradenitis Suppurativa, individuals and healthcare providers can take proactive steps to mitigate the development and progression of the condition.

For those with a genetic predisposition or family history of HS, regular monitoring and early intervention can be crucial in preventing or delaying the onset of the disease. This may involve regular skin examinations, prompt treatment of any suspicious lesions, and close collaboration with healthcare providers to implement preventive measures.

Similarly, for individuals who are overweight or obese, weight management through a healthy diet and regular physical activity can be an important preventive strategy, as it may help to reduce the chronic inflammation and skin-to-skin friction that contribute to the development of HS.

For those who smoke, cessation of tobacco use can significantly reduce the risk of developing Hidradenitis Suppurativa and may also slow the progression of the condition.

Addressing and managing stress through various coping mechanisms, such as mindfulness practices, counseling, or stress-reduction techniques, may also be a valuable preventive measure, as chronic stress has been linked to the exacerbation of HS.

Personalized Management Approaches

Understanding the individual risk factors and triggers for Hidradenitis Suppurativa also allows for the development of more personalized management strategies. By working closely with healthcare providers to identify the specific elements that contribute to their HS, individuals can tailor their treatment plans, lifestyle modifications, and self-care routines to address their unique needs.

For example, individuals with a strong genetic predisposition may require more proactive, aggressive treatment approaches, including the use of targeted therapies or early surgical interventions, to mitigate the risk of disease progression.

Similarly, those who are overweight or obese may benefit from a comprehensive management plan that incorporates weight loss strategies, in addition to traditional HS treatments, to address the underlying inflammatory processes.

Individuals who smoke or experience high levels of stress may need to prioritize smoking cessation and stress management as part of their HS management plan, in conjunction with other therapeutic interventions.

By empowering individuals with Hidradenitis Suppurativa to recognize and address the unique risk factors and triggers associated with their condition, we can enable them to take a more active role in their healthcare, leading to improved outcomes, better quality of life, and greater self-efficacy in managing this complex and often debilitating skin disease.

Conclusion

Hidradenitis Suppurativa is a multifactorial condition, with a complex interplay of genetic, hormonal, and environmental risk factors contributing to its development and progression. Understanding these various influencing elements is crucial for both the prevention and management of this chronic, recurrent skin condition.

Genetic predisposition, hormonal fluctuations, and environmental factors, such as obesity, smoking, and chronic stress, have all been identified as significant risk factors for Hidradenitis Suppurativa. By recognizing these contributing elements, individuals living with HS can take proactive steps to mitigate the development and exacerbation of their condition, working closely with healthcare providers to implement personalized prevention and management strategies.

Empowering individuals with HS to identify and address their unique risk factors and triggers is a fundamental step in improving their overall health, quality of life, and long-term outcomes. This knowledge, in combination with a comprehensive understanding of the symptoms and stages of Hidradenitis Suppurativa, will serve as a crucial foundation as we explore the various diagnostic and treatment approaches in the chapters to come.

CHAPTER 4

I mpact of Hidradenitis Suppurativa on Quality of Life

Addressing the Multifaceted Burden of a Chronic Skin Condition

Hidradenitis Suppurativa (HS) is a chronic, debilitating skin condition that extends far beyond the physical symptoms experienced by those affected. This complex disease can have a profound impact on an individual's emotional, social, and overall quality of life, often leading to a significant burden that extends across multiple aspects of their daily lives.

In this chapter, we will delve into the multifaceted impact of Hidradenitis Suppurativa, examining the physical, emotional, and social challenges faced by individuals living with this condition. We will explore the ways in which HS can impair an individual's ability to engage in daily activities, maintain relationships, and pursue personal and professional goals. Additionally, we will discuss the stigma and misunderstanding that often surrounds HS, as well as the associated comorbidities that can further exacerbate the burden of this chronic skin disease.

By gaining a comprehensive understanding of the wide-ranging impact of Hidradenitis Suppurativa, we can better equip individuals affected by HS, their loved ones, and healthcare providers to address the holistic needs of those living with this debilitating condition. This knowledge will serve as a crucial foundation for developing more effective, patient-centered approaches to the management and support of individuals with Hidradenitis Suppurativa.

Physical Burden and Functional Impairment

At the core of the impact of Hidradenitis Suppurativa is the physical burden experienced by those living with the condition. The hallmark symptoms of HS, including painful lesions, abscesses, and sinus tracts, can significantly impair an individual's ability to perform even the most basic daily activities.

The chronic, recurrent nature of Hidradenitis Suppurativa means that individuals often experience cycles of flare-ups and remissions, with periods of relative calm punctuated by sudden, debilitating outbreaks. During these flare-ups, the pain, discomfort, and physical limitations imposed by the condition can be truly overwhelming, making it challenging for individuals to engage in activities such as getting dressed, using the bathroom, or participating in physical exercise.

The physical symptoms of HS can also lead to functional impairment, as the pain and discomfort associated with the condition can make it difficult for individuals to maintain their usual levels of mobility, dexterity, and overall physical functioning. This can have a cascading impact on an individual's ability to perform work-related tasks, manage their personal care, or participate in recreational and social activities.

Furthermore, the chronic nature of Hidradenitis Suppurativa and the potential for scarring and disfigurement can lead to long-term physical limitations and disabilities, further exacerbating the burden of the condition and the challenges faced by those living with it.

Emotional and Psychological Impact

In addition to the physical burden, Hidradenitis Suppurativa can also have a significant emotional and psychological impact on individuals affected by the condition. The constant pain, disfigurement, and social stigma associated with HS can lead to a wide range of mental health challenges, including depression, anxiety, and low self-esteem.

Many individuals with Hidradenitis Suppurativa report feeling misunderstood, stigmatized, and unsupported by healthcare providers and their own social circles. The visible nature of the lesions and the sometimes-unpleasant odor associated with the condition can contribute to feelings of embarrassment, shame, and social isolation.

The emotional toll of HS can be particularly pronounced during an individual's formative years, when social connections and self-image are of great importance. The impact of the condition on an individual's mental health and overall well-being can have far-reaching consequences, affecting their ability to maintain healthy interpersonal relationships, pursue educational or career goals, and engage in activities that bring them joy and fulfillment.

The psychological burden of Hidradenitis Suppurativa can also lead to a vicious cycle, where the emotional distress exacerbates the physical symptoms of the condition and vice versa. This interplay between the physical and emotional aspects of HS highlights the need for a holistic, multidisciplinary approach to the management of this chronic skin disease.

Social and Occupational Implications

The physical and emotional challenges posed by Hidradenitis Suppurativa can also have significant social and occupational implications for those affected by the condition.

Social Functioning and Relationships
    The recurrent nature of HS flare-ups and the associated physical symptoms and disfigurement can make it challenging for individuals to participate in

social activities, maintain existing relationships, and develop new connections.

The pain, discomfort, and self-consciousness experienced during HS flare-ups can lead to social withdrawal, as individuals may avoid social situations to prevent embarrassment or discomfort. This can further contribute to feelings of isolation and exacerbate the emotional burden of the condition.

Moreover, the stigma and misunderstanding surrounding Hidradenitis Suppurativa can make it difficult for individuals to openly discuss their condition with friends, family members, or potential romantic partners, leading to a sense of isolation and a lack of understanding and support.

Occupational Challenges

The physical limitations and frequent absences from work or school associated with Hidradenitis Suppurativa can have significant occupational and educational implications for those affected by the condition.

The recurrent nature of HS flare-ups and the inability to perform certain tasks due to pain or physical limitations can make it challenging for individuals to maintain steady employment or academic progress. This can lead to financial insecurity, difficulties in career advancement, and feelings of professional and personal stagnation.

Moreover, the stigma and misunderstanding surrounding HS can make it difficult for individuals to openly discuss their condition with employers or academic institutions, potentially leading to discrimination, lack of accommodations, or even job loss.

The occupational challenges faced by individuals with Hidradenitis Suppurativa can have long-lasting consequences, affecting their financial stability, career trajectories, and overall sense of purpose and fulfillment.

Comorbidities and Associated Conditions

Hidradenitis Suppurativa is not an isolated condition, and it is often accompanied by a range of comorbidities and associated conditions that can further exacerbate the burden experienced by those living with the disease.

Metabolic Disorders

Individuals with Hidradenitis Suppurativa have a higher risk of developing metabolic disorders, such as obesity, type 2 diabetes, and metabolic syndrome. These comorbidities can not only contribute to the development and progression of HS but also increase the overall physical and emotional burden experienced by those affected.

The interplay between HS and metabolic disorders can create a self-perpetuating cycle, where the chronic inflammation and physical limitations associated with the skin condition can lead to weight gain and increased risk of metabolic disorders, which in turn can worsen the symptoms of HS.

Addressing these comorbidities through a comprehensive, holistic approach to management is crucial for improving the overall health and well-being of individuals living with Hidradenitis Suppurativa.

Psychiatric Conditions

The emotional and psychological impact of Hidradenitis Suppurativa can also increase the risk of developing psychiatric conditions, such as depression and anxiety.

The constant pain, disfigurement, and social stigma associated with HS can lead to a range of mental health challenges, including low self-esteem, social isolation, and feelings of hopelessness. These mental health issues can further exacerbate the burden of the condition, creating a vicious cycle that can be difficult to break.

Recognizing and addressing the mental health needs of individuals with Hidradenitis Suppurativa is essential for providing comprehensive, patient-centered care and improving their overall quality of life.

Inflammatory Bowel Diseases

There is a well-established link between Hidradenitis Suppurativa and inflammatory bowel diseases (IBDs), such as Crohn's disease and ulcerative colitis. Individuals with HS have a higher risk of developing IBDs, and the presence of these comorbidities can significantly impact the management and outcomes of both conditions.

The shared underlying inflammatory mechanisms and the potential for overlapping symptoms between HS and IBDs can make it challenging to diagnose and manage these conditions effectively. Healthcare providers must be vigilant in identifying and addressing any potential comorbidities to ensure the best possible outcomes for individuals living with Hidradenitis Suppurativa.

Recognizing and Addressing the Holistic Impact of HS

The multifaceted impact of Hidradenitis Suppurativa, encompassing physical, emotional, social, and occupational domains, highlights the need for a comprehensive, holistic approach to the management and support of individuals living with this chronic skin condition.

Healthcare providers, policymakers, and society as a whole must recognize the significant burden borne by those affected by HS and work towards developing more effective strategies for addressing their diverse needs. This includes:

1. Promoting Awareness and Understanding: Increasing public and healthcare provider awareness about the impact of Hidradenitis Suppurativa can help to destigmatize the condition and improve access to appropriate care

and support.

2. Implementing Multidisciplinary Care: A collaborative, multidisciplinary approach involving dermatologists, primary care providers, mental health professionals, and other specialists is essential for addressing the physical, emotional, and social needs of individuals with HS.

3. Advocating for Improved Access to Care: Ensuring that individuals with Hidradenitis Suppurativa have access to timely, comprehensive, and affordable healthcare services is crucial for improving their overall quality of life.

4. Fostering Support Networks and Community Engagement: Facilitating the development of support groups, online communities, and other resources can help individuals with HS feel less isolated and empower them to advocate for their needs.

5. Addressing Occupational and Educational Challenges: Collaborating with employers, schools, and policymakers to implement accommodations, flexible schedules, and anti-discrimination policies can help individuals with HS maintain their professional and educational pursuits.

6. Prioritizing Mental Health and Emotional Well-being: Integrating mental health support, counseling, and stress management techniques into the overall management of Hidradenitis Suppurativa is crucial for improving the holistic well-being of those affected.

By recognizing and addressing the multifaceted impact of Hidradenitis Suppurativa, we can work towards a future where individuals living with this chronic skin condition are empowered, supported, and able to achieve their full potential, despite the challenges they face.

Conclusion

Hidradenitis Suppurativa is a complex, chronic skin condition that extends far beyond the physical symptoms experienced by those affected. This debilitating disease can have a profound impact on an individual's emotional, social, and overall quality of life, leading to a significant burden that permeates multiple aspects of their daily lives.

From the physical limitations and functional impairment caused by the condition's hallmark symptoms to the emotional distress and social isolation, Hidradenitis Suppurativa can profoundly compromise an individual's ability to engage in activities, maintain relationships, and pursue personal and professional goals.

Moreover, the comorbidities and associated conditions that often accompany HS, such as metabolic disorders, psychiatric conditions, and inflammatory bowel diseases, can further exacerbate the overall burden experienced by those living with this chronic skin condition.

Recognizing and addressing the holistic impact of Hidradenitis Suppurativa is essential for providing comprehensive, patient-centered care and support. By promoting awareness, implementing multidisciplinary approaches, advocating for improved access to care, and prioritizing mental health and emotional well-being, we can work towards a future where individuals with HS are empowered, supported, and able to thrive despite the challenges they face.

As we continue our exploration of Hidradenitis Suppurativa, this understanding of the wide-ranging impact of the condition will serve as a critical foundation for developing more effective, holistic strategies for the diagnosis, management, and support of those living with this debilitating skin disease.

CHAPTER 5

D iagnosis and Assessment of Hidradenitis Suppurativa

Navigating the Path to Accurate Identification and Evaluation

Accurate diagnosis and comprehensive assessment are essential first steps in the effective management of Hidradenitis Suppurativa (HS). This chronic, recurrent skin condition can often be challenging to identify, as its clinical presentation can mimic other dermatological disorders, leading to potential misdiagnosis or delayed recognition.

In this chapter, we will explore the various diagnostic techniques and assessment methods used to identify and evaluate Hidradenitis Suppurativa, empowering both individuals living with HS and healthcare providers to navigate the path towards accurate diagnosis and appropriate treatment planning.

Recognizing the Hallmark Signs and Symptoms

The initial step in diagnosing Hidradenitis Suppurativa is to recognize the condition's hallmark signs and symptoms. As discussed in previous chapters, the primary manifestations of HS include:

1. Painful, recurrent lesions and abscesses: The development of painful, inflamed boils or nodules, often in the apocrine sweat gland-bearing areas of

the body, such as the armpits, groin, and buttocks.

2. Sinus tract formation: The progression of lesions into interconnected, draining tunnels or fistulas within the affected skin.

3. Chronic, recurrent nature: The cyclical pattern of flare-ups and remissions that characterize the disease.

4. Odor and drainage: The presence of foul-smelling discharge or drainage from the affected areas.

By being aware of these key clinical features, healthcare providers can begin to suspect the presence of Hidradenitis Suppurativa and initiate a more comprehensive evaluation.

Physical Examination Techniques

The physical examination is a crucial component of the diagnostic process for Hidradenitis Suppurativa. Healthcare providers, typically dermatologists, will perform a thorough examination of the affected areas, looking for the characteristic lesions, abscesses, and sinus tracts associated with the condition.

During the physical examination, the provider may:

1. Palpate the affected areas to assess for the presence of tender nodules, abscesses, or sinus tracts.
2. Visually inspect the skin for the presence of boils, papules, or draining fistulas.
3. Evaluate the extent and distribution of the lesions, as well as any associated scarring or sinus tract formation.
4. Assess the severity of the condition based on established clinical staging

systems, such as the Hurley Staging System.

The physical examination can provide valuable insight into the stage and severity of the Hidradenitis Suppurativa, guiding the next steps in the diagnostic and treatment process.

Diagnostic Imaging and Laboratory Tests

In addition to the physical examination, healthcare providers may utilize various diagnostic imaging and laboratory tests to support the diagnosis of Hidradenitis Suppurativa and rule out other potential conditions.

Imaging Techniques

Diagnostic imaging can play a crucial role in the assessment of Hidradenitis Suppurativa, particularly in identifying the extent of disease involvement and the presence of sinus tracts or deeper tissue involvement.

Common imaging modalities used in the evaluation of HS include:

1. Ultrasound: This non-invasive imaging technique can help visualize the depth and extent of lesions, as well as the presence of sinus tracts or abscesses.

2. Magnetic Resonance Imaging (MRI): MRI can provide detailed, high-resolution images of the affected areas, enabling the identification of deep tissue involvement, fistulas, and the extent of the disease.

3. Computed Tomography (CT) Scan: CT scans may be utilized to assess for the presence of any underlying bone or soft tissue involvement.

The information provided by these imaging techniques can assist healthcare providers in accurately staging the disease, planning appropriate treatment strategies, and monitoring the response to therapy.

Laboratory Tests

While there is no single laboratory test that can definitively diagnose Hidradenitis Suppurativa, healthcare providers may order a variety of tests to support the clinical diagnosis and rule out other potential conditions.

Common laboratory tests that may be performed include:

1. Bacterial cultures: To identify any secondary bacterial infections within the lesions or sinus tracts.
2. Inflammatory markers: Such as C-reactive protein (CRP) or erythrocyte sedimentation rate (ESR), which may be elevated in individuals with HS.
3. Hormonal assessments: To evaluate potential hormonal imbalances that may contribute to the development or progression of the condition.

The results of these laboratory tests, in conjunction with the clinical presentation and diagnostic imaging findings, can help healthcare providers refine the diagnosis and guide the development of a comprehensive management plan.

Differential Diagnosis and Exclusion of Other Conditions

One of the challenges in diagnosing Hidradenitis Suppurativa is that its clinical presentation can often resemble other dermatological conditions, leading to potential misdiagnosis or delayed recognition of the condition.

Healthcare providers must carefully consider the differential diagnosis and systematically exclude other potential conditions that may present with similar signs and symptoms, such as:

1. Acne: Particularly the inflammatory, nodular, and cystic forms of acne,

which can share some overlapping features with HS.

2. Folliculitis: Inflammation and infection of the hair follicles, which can manifest as boils or abscesses in the affected areas.

3. Furuncles and carbuncles: Severe, deep-seated infections of the hair follicles, which can be mistaken for HS lesions.

4. Inflammatory bowel diseases (IBDs): Conditions like Crohn's disease or ulcerative colitis, which can sometimes present with skin manifestations that resemble HS.

5. Pilonidal cysts: Localized, inflamed cysts that can develop in the gluteal cleft, potentially mimicking the appearance of HS lesions.

To differentiate Hidradenitis Suppurativa from these other conditions, healthcare providers may need to consider a combination of the patient's medical history, physical examination findings, diagnostic test results, and, in some cases, a skin biopsy for histological analysis.

Establishing an accurate diagnosis is crucial, as it enables the development of an appropriate treatment plan and helps to avoid potentially inappropriate or ineffective interventions.

Utilizing Clinical Staging Systems

To facilitate the assessment and management of Hidradenitis Suppurativa, healthcare providers often utilize standardized clinical staging systems, such as the Hurley Staging System, to categorize the severity of the condition.

The Hurley Staging System classifies HS into three distinct stages based on the clinical presentation and extent of disease involvement:

1. Hurley Stage I (Mild): Characterized by the presence of isolated, single or multiple, abscess formations without sinus tracts or scarring.

2. Hurley Stage II (Moderate): Marked by recurrent abscesses, with widely separated, single or multiple, well-defined lesions and the formation of sinus tracts and scarring.

3. Hurley Stage III (Severe): Defined by the presence of diffuse or near-diffuse involvement, with multiple, interconnected sinus tracts and abscesses, as well as substantial scarring.

By categorizing the stage of Hidradenitis Suppurativa, healthcare providers can better assess the severity of the condition, guide the selection of appropriate treatment modalities, and monitor the patient's response to therapy over time.

It is important to note that the Hurley Staging System provides a framework for understanding the progression of HS, but it is not a perfect predictor of an individual's disease course or response to treatment. The condition can be dynamic, with individuals potentially experiencing fluctuations between stages or exhibiting a mix of clinical features from different stages.

Comprehensive Assessment and Personalized Care

Ultimately, the diagnosis and assessment of Hidradenitis Suppurativa require a comprehensive, multifaceted approach that considers the individual's medical history, clinical presentation, diagnostic test results, and the impact of the condition on their overall well-being.

By taking a holistic, patient-centered approach to the evaluation of HS, healthcare providers can develop a thorough understanding of the condition's manifestations, underlying causes, and the unique challenges faced by each individual. This, in turn, enables the development of personalized management strategies that address the physical, emotional, and social needs of those living with Hidradenitis Suppurativa.

Key components of a comprehensive assessment for Hidradenitis Suppurativa may include:

1. Detailed medical history: Gathering information about the onset, progression, and impact of the condition, as well as any associated comorbidities or triggers.

2. Thorough physical examination: Assessing the extent, severity, and pattern of lesions, as well as any evidence of sinus tract formation or scarring.

3. Diagnostic testing: Utilizing appropriate imaging modalities and laboratory analyses to support the diagnosis and guide treatment planning.

4. Assessment of quality of life: Evaluating the physical, emotional, and social impact of the condition on the individual's overall well-being and functioning.

5. Collaborative decision-making: Engaging the individual in the assessment process and incorporating their preferences and goals into the management plan.

By adopting a holistic, patient-centered approach to the diagnosis and assessment of Hidradenitis Suppurativa, healthcare providers can empower individuals living with this chronic skin condition to play an active role in their care, ultimately leading to improved outcomes and a better quality of life.

Conclusion

Accurate diagnosis and comprehensive assessment are essential first steps in the effective management of Hidradenitis Suppurativa. This complex, recurrent skin condition can present a challenge for healthcare providers, as its clinical manifestations can often resemble other dermatological disorders, leading to potential misdiagnosis or delayed recognition.

To navigate the path towards accurate identification and evaluation of Hidradenitis Suppurativa, healthcare providers must be equipped with a thorough understanding of the hallmark signs and symptoms of the condition, as well as the various diagnostic techniques and assessment methods available.

By leveraging physical examination techniques, diagnostic imaging, and laboratory tests, healthcare providers can work to confirm the diagnosis, rule out other potential conditions, and establish the stage and severity of the individual's Hidradenitis Suppurativa. The utilization of standardized clinical staging systems, such as the Hurley Staging System, can further enhance the assessment process and guide the development of personalized treatment strategies.

Ultimately, the diagnosis and assessment of Hidradenitis Suppurativa require a comprehensive, patient-centered approach that considers the individual's unique medical history, clinical presentation, and the impact of the condition on their overall well-being. By adopting this holistic perspective, healthcare providers can empower individuals living with HS to play an active role in their care, leading to improved outcomes and a better quality of life.

As we continue our exploration of Hidradenitis Suppurativa, this understanding of the diagnostic and assessment process will serve as a crucial foundation for the development and implementation of effective treatment strategies, which will be the focus of the chapters to come.

CHAPTER 6

Conservative Treatment Approaches for Hidradenitis Suppurativa

Optimizing Outcomes through Targeted, Evidence-Based Interventions

The management of Hidradenitis Suppurativa (HS) often begins with conservative treatment approaches, which aim to provide symptom relief, prevent disease progression, and improve the overall quality of life for individuals living with this chronic, recurrent skin condition.

In this chapter, we will explore the various conservative treatment options available for Hidradenitis Suppurativa, including topical medications, oral therapies, and lifestyle modifications. By understanding the mechanisms of action, efficacy, and appropriate application of these interventions, healthcare providers and individuals with HS can work collaboratively to develop personalized treatment plans that address the diverse needs and preferences of those affected by this debilitating condition.

The Role of Topical Medications

Topical treatments are often the first-line approach in the management of mild to moderate Hidradenitis Suppurativa. These medications are applied directly to the affected areas of the skin and can help to address the localized inflammation, infection, and other symptoms associated with the condition.

Topical Antibiotics

Topical antibiotics are commonly used in the treatment of Hidradenitis Suppurativa, as they can help to control secondary bacterial infections that may arise within the lesions and sinus tracts.

Some of the commonly prescribed topical antibiotics for HS include:
- Clindamycin: A lincosamide antibiotic that has demonstrated efficacy in reducing the number and severity of HS lesions.
- Erythromycin: A macrolide antibiotic that can be used as an alternative to clindamycin.
- Mupirocin: A topical antibiotic that has been shown to have a positive impact on HS symptoms.

The mechanism of action of these topical antibiotics involves the reduction of bacterial load, which can help to prevent the progression of lesions and the development of secondary infections.

Topical Retinoids

Topical retinoids, such as adapalene and tazarotene, have also been explored as treatment options for Hidradenitis Suppurativa. These medications work by modulating the follicular keratinization process, which can help to prevent the obstruction of hair follicles and the subsequent development of lesions.

Studies have suggested that topical retinoids may be particularly effective in the early stages of HS, where they can help to prevent the progression of the condition and potentially delay the need for more advanced interventions.

Topical Anti-Inflammatory Agents

In addition to antibiotics and retinoids, topical anti-inflammatory agents, such as glucocorticoids (corticosteroids) and calcineurin inhibitors, have been used to manage the localized inflammation associated with Hidradenitis Suppurativa.

Topical corticosteroids, for example, can help to reduce swelling, redness, and pain within the affected areas. However, the long-term use of these medications may be limited due to potential side effects, such as skin thinning and disruption of the skin barrier.

Calcineurin inhibitors, such as tacrolimus and pimecrolimus, have also been explored as topical treatments for HS, as they can help to modulate the immune response and reduce inflammation without the same risks associated with corticosteroids.

When using topical medications for Hidradenitis Suppurativa, it is essential to follow the instructions provided by healthcare providers carefully, as the appropriate application and duration of use can vary depending on the specific medication and the individual's response to treatment.

Oral Therapies for Hidradenitis Suppurativa

In cases where topical treatments are not sufficient or when the disease is more severe, healthcare providers may recommend the use of oral therapies to manage Hidradenitis Suppurativa.

Oral Antibiotics

Systemic antibiotic therapy is a common approach in the management of moderate to severe HS. The selection of the appropriate oral antibiotic is typically based on the severity of the condition, the presence of any secondary infections, and the individual's response to previous treatments.

Some of the commonly prescribed oral antibiotics for Hidradenitis Suppurativa include:
- Clindamycin: Often used in combination with rifampicin for its synergistic effects.
- Tetracyclines (e.g., doxycycline, minocycline): Known for their anti-inflammatory properties in addition to their antimicrobial effects.

- Macrolides (e.g., erythromycin, azithromycin): Used as alternatives or in combination with other antibiotics.

The duration of oral antibiotic therapy for HS can vary, with some individuals requiring long-term, continuous treatment to maintain disease control and prevent recurrence.

Hormonal Therapies

Given the potential role of hormonal factors in the development and progression of Hidradenitis Suppurativa, hormonal therapies have been explored as treatment options for the condition.

Oral contraceptives, for instance, have been used to manage HS in women, as they can help to regulate hormonal fluctuations and potentially reduce disease activity. Similarly, anti-androgen medications, such as spironolactone, have been investigated for their ability to target the hormonal imbalances that may contribute to the pathogenesis of HS.

It is important to note that the use of hormonal therapies for Hidradenitis Suppurativa is often an "off-label" application, as these medications are not specifically approved for the treatment of HS. Healthcare providers must carefully weigh the potential benefits and risks of hormonal interventions, particularly in the context of each individual's medical history and preferences.

Immunomodulatory Agents

In addition to antibiotics and hormonal therapies, certain immunomodulatory agents have been investigated for their potential in the management of Hidradenitis Suppurativa. These medications work by targeting specific aspects of the immune system to reduce inflammation and disease activity.

Examples of oral immunomodulatory agents used in the treatment of HS include:

- Apremilast: A phosphodiesterase-4 (PDE4) inhibitor that has demonstrated efficacy in reducing HS symptoms.

- Methotrexate: A disease-modifying antirheumatic drug (DMARD) that can help to manage the inflammatory processes underlying HS.

- Acitretin: A retinoid medication that has been used to target the follicular occlusion and hyperkeratosis associated with the condition.

The use of these immunomodulatory agents often requires close monitoring by healthcare providers, as they can be associated with potential side effects and may interact with other medications the individual is taking.

Lifestyle Modifications and Wound Care

In addition to topical and oral therapies, lifestyle modifications and proper wound care are essential components of a comprehensive management plan for Hidradenitis Suppurativa.

Weight Management

As discussed in previous chapters, obesity is a well-established risk factor for Hidradenitis Suppurativa. Therefore, weight loss and maintaining a healthy body weight can be an important strategy in the management of HS.

Through a combination of dietary changes, increased physical activity, and potential medical interventions (e.g., bariatric surgery), individuals with HS who are overweight or obese can work to reduce the chronic inflammation and skin-to-skin friction that may contribute to the development and progression of their condition.

Smoking Cessation

Smoking has been identified as a significant risk factor for Hidradenitis Suppurativa, and the cessation of tobacco use can have a positive impact on the course of the disease.

Healthcare providers should strongly encourage individuals with HS who smoke to quit, as doing so may help to reduce the severity of symptoms, prevent disease progression, and potentially improve the efficacy of other treatment interventions.

Stress Management

While the relationship between stress and Hidradenitis Suppurativa is not fully understood, evidence suggests that chronic stress may play a role in triggering or exacerbating HS flare-ups.

Incorporating stress management techniques, such as mindfulness practices, relaxation exercises, and counseling, into the overall management plan for HS can help to mitigate the impact of stress on the individual's physical and emotional well-being.

Proper Wound Care

During HS flare-ups, the proper care and management of the affected areas are essential to prevent the development of secondary infections, promote healing, and reduce the risk of complications.

This may involve:
- Gentle cleansing of the lesions and sinus tracts
- Application of topical antiseptic or antimicrobial agents
- Appropriate dressing and bandaging techniques
- Avoidance of irritation or trauma to the affected areas

By educating individuals with Hidradenitis Suppurativa on proper wound care practices and empowering them to take an active role in the management of their condition, healthcare providers can help to improve outcomes and prevent further disease progression.

Integrating Conservative Approaches into a Comprehensive Management Plan

The conservative treatment approaches discussed in this chapter, including topical medications, oral therapies, and lifestyle modifications, are often the initial steps in the management of Hidradenitis Suppurativa. However, it is important to recognize that the efficacy of these interventions can vary among individuals, and the condition's chronic, recurrent nature may require a more comprehensive, multifaceted approach to care.

Healthcare providers should work collaboratively with individuals living with Hidradenitis Suppurativa to develop personalized treatment plans that address the unique needs and preferences of each patient. This may involve a combination of conservative approaches, with the potential for escalation to more advanced interventions, such as intralesional injections, biologic therapies, or surgical treatments, if the condition does not respond adequately to the initial management strategies.

Moreover, the integration of conservative treatments into a holistic management plan should also consider the impact of HS on the individual's physical, emotional, and social well-being. By addressing the multifaceted burden of the condition and supporting the individual's overall quality of life, healthcare providers can help to maximize the effectiveness of the chosen interventions and empower those living with Hidradenitis Suppurativa to actively participate in their own care.

Conclusion

Conservative treatment approaches, including topical medications, oral therapies, and lifestyle modifications, play a crucial role in the management of Hidradenitis Suppurativa. These interventions aim to provide symptom relief, prevent disease progression, and improve the overall quality of life for individuals living with this chronic, recurrent skin condition.

By understanding the mechanisms of action, efficacy, and appropriate application of these conservative treatment options, healthcare providers and individuals with HS can work collaboratively to develop personalized management plans that address the diverse needs and preferences of those affected by this debilitating condition.

The integration of conservative approaches into a comprehensive, multi-faceted management strategy is essential, as the chronic nature of Hidradenitis Suppurativa may require a combination of interventions to achieve optimal outcomes. Additionally, the consideration of the individual's physical, emotional, and social well-being is crucial in ensuring that the chosen treatment plan effectively addresses the holistic impact of the condition.

As we continue our exploration of Hidradenitis Suppurativa, the understanding of conservative treatment approaches will serve as a foundation for the subsequent chapters, which will delve into more advanced interventions, such as intralesional injections, biologic therapies, and surgical treatments, as well as the evolving landscape of HS management.

CHAPTER 7

A dvanced Treatment Options for Hidradenitis Suppurativa

Harnessing Innovative Therapies to Manage a Chronic, Debilitating Condition

While conservative treatment approaches, as discussed in the previous chapter, play a crucial role in the management of Hidradenitis Suppurativa (HS), there are instances where more advanced interventions may be necessary to effectively control the condition and improve the overall quality of life for individuals affected by this chronic, recurrent skin disease.

In this chapter, we will explore the various advanced treatment options available for Hidradenitis Suppurativa, including intralesional injections, biologic therapies, and surgical interventions. By understanding the mechanisms of action, efficacy, and appropriate application of these more specialized treatment modalities, healthcare providers and individuals with HS can work collaboratively to develop personalized management strategies that address the complex and often challenging nature of this debilitating condition.

Intralesional Injections

Intralesional injections, or the direct injection of therapeutic agents into the affected lesions, have emerged as a valuable treatment option for individuals with Hidradenitis Suppurativa, particularly in cases where topical and oral therapies have proven insufficient.

Corticosteroid Injections

One of the most commonly utilized intralesional treatments for HS is the injection of corticosteroids, such as triamcinolone acetonide, directly into the affected lesions or abscesses.

The mechanism of action of these intralesional corticosteroid injections involves the localized reduction of inflammation, which can help to alleviate the pain, swelling, and progression of the HS lesions. Additionally, the targeted delivery of the corticosteroid to the affected areas can minimize the systemic absorption and potential side effects associated with oral or topical corticosteroid use.

Studies have shown that intralesional corticosteroid injections can be an effective adjunctive therapy for individuals with Hidradenitis Suppurativa, particularly in the management of localized, recurrent lesions or abscesses. However, the long-term use of these injections may be limited due to the potential for skin discoloration, thinning, or other adverse effects.

Intralesional Biologics

In recent years, the use of intralesional biologic agents, such as adalimumab (a tumor necrosis factor-alpha [TNF-α] inhibitor), has been explored as a treatment option for Hidradenitis Suppurativa.

The rationale behind the use of intralesional biologics in HS is to target the specific inflammatory pathways and cytokines that play a key role in the pathogenesis of the condition. By delivering the biologic agent directly to the affected lesions, healthcare providers can potentially achieve a higher local concentration of the therapeutic agent, while minimizing the systemic exposure and associated side effects.

Preliminary studies have suggested that intralesional injections of biologics, such as adalimumab, can be an effective and well-tolerated treatment approach for individuals with Hidradenitis Suppurativa, particularly in cases where systemic biologic therapies have been unsuccessful or not well-tolerated.

It is important to note that the use of intralesional biologics for the treatment of HS is still considered an off-label application, and further research is necessary to establish the long-term efficacy and safety of this treatment modality.

Biologic Therapies

The advent of biologic medications, which target specific components of the immune system, has revolutionized the treatment landscape for Hidradenitis Suppurativa. These innovative therapies have emerged as a game-changing option for individuals with moderate to severe HS who have not responded adequately to conservative or traditional treatment approaches.

Tumor Necrosis Factor-Alpha (TNF-α) Inhibitors
    One of the most extensively studied and utilized biologic therapies for Hidradenitis Suppurativa is the class of tumor necrosis factor-alpha (TNF-α) inhibitors. These medications work by blocking the action of the pro-inflammatory cytokine TNF-α, which plays a central role in the pathogenesis of HS.

Examples of TNF-α inhibitors approved for the treatment of Hidradenitis Suppurativa include:
    - Adalimumab
    - Infliximab
    - Etanercept

These biologic agents have demonstrated significant efficacy in the management of moderate to severe HS, with studies showing improvements in lesion counts, pain, and overall quality of life for individuals receiving these treatments.

Interleukin (IL) Inhibitors

In addition to TNF-α inhibitors, biologic therapies that target other key inflammatory mediators, such as interleukins (ILs), have also been explored for the treatment of Hidradenitis Suppurativa.

One example is the IL-17 inhibitor, secukinumab, which has shown promising results in the management of HS. By inhibiting the action of IL-17, a cytokine involved in the inflammatory cascade, secukinumab can help to reduce the underlying inflammation and potentially improve the clinical symptoms of the condition.

Similarly, the IL-12/23 inhibitor, ustekinumab, has also been investigated as a biologic therapy for Hidradenitis Suppurativa, with studies suggesting that it may be an effective treatment option for individuals with moderate to severe disease.

The use of biologic therapies in the management of Hidradenitis Suppurativa represents a significant advancement in the field, as these targeted interventions can provide a more effective and potentially long-lasting solution for individuals struggling with this chronic, debilitating condition.

However, it is important to note that the use of biologic agents is often reserved for individuals with moderate to severe HS who have not responded adequately to conservative or traditional treatment approaches. Additionally, the long-term safety and potential side effects associated with these medications require close monitoring and collaboration between healthcare providers and individuals with HS.

Surgical Interventions

In cases where conservative and advanced medical therapies have been insufficient in controlling the symptoms and progression of Hidradenitis Suppurativa, surgical interventions may be considered as part of a comprehensive management approach.

Surgical treatments for HS aim to address the underlying pathological processes, such as follicular occlusion and chronic inflammation, by physically removing or modifying the affected areas of the skin and subcutaneous tissue.

Wide Local Excision

One of the most commonly performed surgical procedures for Hidradenitis Suppurativa is wide local excision, also known as surgical excision or deroofing.

This approach involves the complete removal of the affected skin and subcutaneous tissue, including any sinus tracts or abscesses, in an effort to eradicate the disease. The resulting wound is then left to heal by secondary intention, meaning that it is allowed to close and heal naturally over time.

Wide local excision has been shown to be an effective treatment option for individuals with severe, recalcitrant Hidradenitis Suppurativa, particularly in cases where the disease is localized to a specific area. However, it is important to note that this procedure can be associated with a significant risk of complications, such as extensive scarring, delayed wound healing, and the potential for recurrence of the disease in the surrounding skin.

Deroofing and Marsupialization

In addition to wide local excision, other surgical techniques, such as deroofing and marsupialization, have also been utilized in the management of Hidradenitis Suppurativa.

Deroofing involves the removal of the roof or the epithelial lining of the sinus tracts, allowing the underlying tissue to granulate and heal. This approach aims to disrupt the cycle of inflammation and recurrence associated with the sinus tract formation.

Marsupialization, on the other hand, is a technique where the roof of the sinus tract is incised and sewn to the surrounding skin, creating a pouch-like structure that can help to prevent the re-epithelialization of the tract and promote healing.

These more targeted surgical interventions may be particularly useful in cases where the disease is localized or when the individual is unable to undergo a more extensive wide local excision procedure.

The selection of the appropriate surgical approach for Hidradenitis Suppurativa should be based on the individual's disease severity, the extent of involvement, and the potential risks and benefits of the intervention. Healthcare providers should work closely with individuals with HS to develop a personalized surgical treatment plan that aligns with their goals, expectations, and overall management strategy.

Integrating Advanced Treatments into a Comprehensive Management Approach

The advanced treatment options discussed in this chapter, including intralesional injections, biologic therapies, and surgical interventions, play a crucial role in the management of Hidradenitis Suppurativa, particularly in cases where conservative approaches have proven insufficient or ineffective.

However, it is important to recognize that the integration of these advanced therapies into a comprehensive management plan should be a collaborative process between healthcare providers and individuals living with HS. The selection and implementation of these interventions should be guided by a thorough evaluation of the individual's disease severity, response to prior treatments, and overall goals and preferences.

In some cases, a stepwise approach may be warranted, where healthcare providers start with more conservative treatments and gradually escalate the intensity of interventions based on the individual's response and the evolution of their condition. This approach can help to ensure that the most appropriate and effective treatment strategies are implemented, while minimizing the potential risks and side effects associated with the more advanced therapies.

Moreover, the integration of advanced treatments should also consider the impact of HS on the individual's physical, emotional, and social well-being. By addressing the holistic needs of those living with this chronic, debilitating condition, healthcare providers can work to optimize the overall effectiveness of the chosen treatment plan and empower individuals to actively participate in their own care.

Ultimately, the successful management of Hidradenitis Suppurativa requires a comprehensive, multidisciplinary approach that incorporates both conservative and advanced treatment modalities, tailored to the unique needs and preferences of each individual. By harnessing the power of innovative therapies and collaborating with individuals living with HS, healthcare providers can work towards improving the quality of life and long-term outcomes for those affected by this challenging skin condition.

Conclusion

The advanced treatment options explored in this chapter, including intralesional injections, biologic therapies, and surgical interventions, have revolutionized the management of Hidradenitis Suppurativa, particularly for individuals with moderate to severe disease who have not responded adequately to conservative treatment approaches.

Intralesional injections, such as those utilizing corticosteroids or biologic agents, can provide targeted, localized therapy for the management of specific lesions or abscesses, while biologic medications that target key inflammatory pathways have demonstrated significant efficacy in improving the clinical symptoms and overall quality of life for individuals living with HS.

In cases where medical therapies have been insufficient, surgical interventions, including wide local excision, deroofing, and marsupialization, may be considered as part of a comprehensive management strategy. These surgical approaches aim to disrupt the underlying pathological processes, such as follicular occlusion and chronic inflammation, that contribute to the development and progression of Hidradenitis Suppurativa.

The integration of these advanced treatment options into a personalized management plan should be a collaborative process between healthcare providers and individuals with HS, taking into account the individual's disease severity, response to prior treatments, and overall goals and preferences. By harnessing the power of innovative therapies and addressing the holistic needs of those living with this chronic, debilitating condition, healthcare providers can work to optimize the long-term outcomes and improve the quality of life for individuals affected by Hidradenitis Suppurativa.

As we continue our exploration of this complex skin condition, the knowledge gained from this chapter on advanced treatment options will serve as a foundation for the subsequent discussions on the management of flare-ups, complications, and the evolving landscape of HS care.

CHAPTER 8

Managing Flare-ups and Complications in Hidradenitis Suppurativa

Navigating the Unpredictable Nature of a Chronic Skin Condition

One of the defining characteristics of Hidradenitis Suppurativa (HS) is its chronic, recurrent nature. Individuals living with this debilitating skin condition often experience cycles of flare-ups and remissions, with sudden, unpredictable outbreaks that can significantly impact their quality of life. Managing these flare-ups and addressing the potential complications associated with HS are essential components of comprehensive care for those affected by this condition.

In this chapter, we will explore strategies for identifying and mitigating the triggers that contribute to HS flare-ups, as well as effective approaches for the acute management of the condition during these exacerbations. Additionally, we will delve into the various complications that can arise in the context of Hidradenitis Suppurativa and discuss long-term management techniques to help individuals living with HS maintain optimal health and well-being despite the chronic, recurrent nature of their condition.

Recognizing and Preventing HS Flare-ups

One of the greatest challenges in managing Hidradenitis Suppurativa is the unpredictable nature of the condition's flare-ups. While the triggers that contribute to these exacerbations are not fully understood, research has identified several potential factors that may precipitate or exacerbate HS symptoms.

Identifying Triggers

Understanding the individual triggers that contribute to HS flare-ups is a crucial first step in the management of this condition. Common potential triggers that have been associated with the onset or worsening of Hidradenitis Suppurativa include:

1. Hormonal fluctuations: Changes in estrogen, testosterone, and other sex hormones can influence the development and progression of HS.
2. Stress and anxiety: Chronic stress has been linked to the exacerbation of HS symptoms, potentially through its effects on the immune system and inflammatory pathways.
3. Friction and irritation: Repetitive mechanical stress or trauma to the affected areas, such as from tight clothing or shaving, can contribute to the development of new lesions.
4. Obesity and weight changes: Fluctuations in body weight, particularly weight gain, have been associated with an increased risk of HS flare-ups.
5. Smoking: The use of tobacco products has been identified as a significant risk factor for the development and worsening of Hidradenitis Suppurativa.
6. Bacterial infections: Secondary bacterial infections within the HS lesions or sinus tracts can lead to acute exacerbations of the condition.

By working closely with healthcare providers to identify their individual triggers, individuals living with Hidradenitis Suppurativa can take proactive steps to avoid or mitigate the factors that may contribute to the onset of flare-ups.

Preventive Strategies

Once the potential triggers have been identified, individuals with Hidradenitis Suppurativa can implement a range of preventive strategies to help minimize the frequency and severity of flare-ups. These strategies may include:

1. Hormone management: For individuals with hormonal influences on their HS, the use of oral contraceptives, anti-androgen medications, or other hormonal therapies may help to stabilize hormonal fluctuations and reduce the risk of flare-ups.
2. Stress management: Incorporating stress-reduction techniques, such as meditation, mindfulness exercises, or counseling, can help to mitigate the impact of chronic stress on HS.
3. Skin care and hygiene: Maintaining proper skin care, including gentle cleansing and the avoidance of irritants, can help to reduce the risk of friction-induced flare-ups.
4. Weight management: For individuals who are overweight or obese, achieving and maintaining a healthy body weight through a combination of diet and exercise can help to reduce the risk of HS flare-ups.
5. Smoking cessation: Quitting smoking and avoiding exposure to tobacco smoke can have a positive impact on the course of Hidradenitis Suppurativa.
6. Early treatment of infections: Prompt recognition and management of any secondary bacterial infections within the HS lesions or sinus tracts can help to prevent the escalation of flare-ups.

By working collaboratively with healthcare providers to identify and address the unique triggers that contribute to their HS flare-ups, individuals can take an active role in managing their condition and improving their overall quality of life.

Acute Management of HS Flare-ups

Despite the implementation of preventive strategies, individuals with Hidradenitis Suppurativa may still experience acute flare-ups of their condition, characterized by the sudden onset or worsening of symptoms. Effective management of these flare-ups is crucial to alleviate the physical and emotional burden experienced by those living with HS.

Symptom-Targeted Interventions

During an HS flare-up, the primary goals of acute management are to address the specific symptoms and complications that arise, such as:

1. Pain management: The use of over-the-counter or prescription pain medications, as well as the application of cold compresses, can help to alleviate the pain associated with HS lesions and abscesses.
2. Reduction of inflammation: Topical or oral anti-inflammatory medications, such as corticosteroids, can help to reduce the swelling and redness of the affected areas.
3. Drainage and wound care: Proper drainage of any abscesses or sinus tracts, followed by appropriate wound care and dressing changes, can help to prevent the development of secondary infections.
4. Antibiotic therapy: The use of topical or systemic antibiotic medications may be necessary to manage any secondary bacterial infections that arise during a flare-up.

Individualized Flare-up Management Plans

To effectively manage acute flare-ups, healthcare providers and individuals with Hidradenitis Suppurativa should work together to develop personalized, step-by-step action plans that can be implemented at the first signs of a flare-up.

These individualized flare-up management plans may include:
   - A list of the individual's typical flare-up symptoms and triggers
   - Instructions for the use of specific medications or interventions to address the acute symptoms
   - Guidance on when to seek additional medical care or escalate the level of treatment
   - Contact information for the healthcare provider or care team

By having a clear, personalized action plan in place, individuals with Hidradenitis Suppurativa can feel empowered to take immediate, appropriate action at the onset of a flare-up, potentially mitigating the severity and duration of the exacerbation.

Collaboration with Healthcare Providers
   Effective management of HS flare-ups requires close collaboration between individuals living with the condition and their healthcare providers. Regular communication, monitoring, and adjustment of the treatment plan are essential to ensure that the individual's needs are being met and that any complications or exacerbations are addressed in a timely and appropriate manner.

Healthcare providers should work with individuals to educate them on the recognition of flare-up symptoms, the implementation of acute interventions, and the appropriate circumstances for seeking additional medical care. This partnership can help to empower individuals with Hidradenitis Suppurativa to take an active role in managing their condition and improve their overall outcomes.

Addressing Potential Complications

Hidradenitis Suppurativa is a complex, chronic condition that can be associated with a range of potential complications, both directly related to the skin manifestations of the disease and indirectly through its impact on an individual's overall health and well-being. Recognizing and addressing these complications is crucial for optimizing the management of Hidradenitis Suppurativa and improving the quality of life for those affected.

Infectious Complications

One of the primary complications associated with Hidradenitis Suppurativa is the development of secondary bacterial infections within the lesions, abscesses, or sinus tracts. These infections can lead to further inflammation, pain, and the potential for the spread of the infection to surrounding areas or even the bloodstream (systemic infection).

Prompt recognition and management of these infectious complications, through the use of topical or systemic antibiotic therapy, is essential to prevent the escalation of the condition and the development of more serious complications.

Fistula Formation

Another potential complication of Hidradenitis Suppurativa is the formation of fistulas, or abnormal connections between the affected skin areas and internal structures, such as the rectum, bladder, or pelvic organs.

Fistulas can lead to persistent drainage, recurrent infections, and significant discomfort for individuals living with HS. In some cases, surgical intervention may be necessary to address the fistula and prevent further complications.

Scarring and Disfigurement

The chronic, recurrent nature of Hidradenitis Suppurativa can result in significant scarring and disfigurement of the affected areas, particularly in cases where the condition is severe or has been present for an extended period.

This scarring can not only be physically uncomfortable but can also have a profound impact on an individual's emotional well-being and self-image. Healthcare providers should work closely with individuals with HS to address the cosmetic and functional consequences of the scarring, potentially through the use of scar management techniques or surgical interventions.

Psychological Complications

The physical and emotional burden of living with Hidradenitis Suppurativa can also lead to the development of various psychological complications, such as depression, anxiety, and low self-esteem.

Addressing the mental health needs of individuals with HS is a crucial component of comprehensive care, as untreated psychological complications can further exacerbate the overall burden of the condition and impair an individual's ability to effectively manage their disease.

Metabolic and Systemic Complications

Hidradenitis Suppurativa has also been associated with an increased risk of certain metabolic and systemic complications, such as obesity, type 2 diabetes, and inflammatory bowel diseases.

These comorbidities can not only contribute to the development and progression of Hidradenitis Suppurativa but can also create a self-perpetuating cycle of poor health outcomes. Addressing these systemic complications through a multidisciplinary approach, involving healthcare providers from various specialties, is essential for optimizing the management of HS and improving the overall well-being of those affected.

Long-term Management Strategies

Given the chronic, recurrent nature of Hidradenitis Suppurativa, the long-term management of the condition is crucial to maintaining optimal health, minimizing the risk of complications, and improving the quality of life for individuals living with this debilitating skin disease.

Continuous Monitoring and Personalized Care

Effective long-term management of Hidradenitis Suppurativa requires continuous monitoring and personalized care from a multidisciplinary team of healthcare providers. This may involve regular follow-up appointments, ongoing evaluation of the individual's disease progression, and the adjustment of treatment strategies as needed.

By maintaining a close partnership with their healthcare providers, individuals with HS can work to identify any changes in their condition, address emerging complications, and proactively implement preventive strategies to mitigate the risk of flare-ups and disease progression.

Comprehensive Disease Management Approach

The long-term management of Hidradenitis Suppurativa should encompass a comprehensive, multifaceted approach that addresses the physical, emotional, and social aspects of the condition. This may include:

1. Ongoing medical treatment: Continued use of topical, oral, or advanced therapies, as well as regular monitoring for disease progression and the development of complications.
2. Psychological support: Access to mental health professionals, support groups, and resources to address the emotional and psychosocial impact of living with HS.
3. Lifestyle modifications: Maintaining a healthy weight, adopting stress-reduction techniques, and avoiding potential triggers to minimize the risk of flare-ups.
4. Wound care and skin management: Proper wound care, hygiene practices, and the use of protective clothing or devices to mitigate the risk of friction and irritation.
5. Surgical interventions: In some cases, the long-term management of HS

may involve the incorporation of surgical treatments, such as excision or deroofing, to address persistent or severe disease.

By implementing a comprehensive, personalized disease management approach, individuals with Hidradenitis Suppurativa can work towards achieving optimal long-term outcomes, minimizing the impact of the condition on their daily lives, and improving their overall quality of life.

Conclusion

Effectively managing the flare-ups and complications associated with Hidradenitis Suppurativa is a crucial aspect of caring for individuals living with this chronic, recurrent skin condition. Understanding the potential triggers that contribute to HS flare-ups and implementing preventive strategies to mitigate these factors can help individuals take a more proactive role in managing their disease.

When acute flare-ups do occur, the implementation of targeted, symptom-based interventions, combined with personalized flare-up management plans, can empower individuals to address the immediate needs and minimize the impact of these exacerbations. Furthermore, recognizing and addressing the potential complications that can arise, such as infections, fistulas, scarring, and psychological or systemic issues, is essential for optimizing the long-term management of Hidradenitis Suppurativa.

Ultimately, the successful long-term management of HS requires a comprehensive, multifaceted approach that addresses the physical, emotional, and social needs of those affected by this debilitating condition. By working collaboratively with healthcare providers, individuals with Hidradenitis Suppurativa can take an active role in their care, implement preventive strategies, and develop the necessary skills and resources to effectively manage the unpredictable nature of their disease.

As we continue our exploration of Hidradenitis Suppurativa, the knowledge gained from this chapter on managing flare-ups and complications will serve as a crucial foundation for understanding the unique considerations and approaches required for specific patient populations, such as children and pregnant individuals, which will be the focus of the following chapters.

CHAPTER 9

Pediatric Hidradenitis Suppurativa

Addressing the Unique Challenges in Caring for Children and Adolescents

While Hidradenitis Suppurativa (HS) is typically considered an adult-onset condition, it can also occur in children and adolescents, presenting unique challenges in diagnosis, management, and overall care. Understanding the distinctive features and considerations associated with pediatric HS is essential for healthcare providers and caregivers to ensure the best possible outcomes for this vulnerable patient population.

In this chapter, we will explore the epidemiology and unique clinical characteristics of Hidradenitis Suppurativa in children and adolescents. We will also delve into the specialized diagnostic and treatment approaches required for this age group, as well as the importance of addressing the psychosocial impacts of the condition and the crucial role of family involvement in the management of pediatric HS.

By gaining a comprehensive understanding of the unique challenges and considerations surrounding Hidradenitis Suppurativa in children and adolescents, we can empower healthcare providers, caregivers, and the young individuals affected to work collaboratively towards improved outcomes and a better quality of life.

Epidemiology and Unique Considerations in Pediatric HS

While Hidradenitis Suppurativa is primarily considered an adult-onset condition, with the highest incidence typically observed in the late teens to early 40s, the disease can also occur in children and adolescents. However, the epidemiology and clinical presentation of HS in the pediatric population may differ in several key ways.

Prevalence and Age of Onset

The exact prevalence of Hidradenitis Suppurativa in children and adolescents is not well-established, as the condition is often underdiagnosed or misdiagnosed in this age group. Nevertheless, studies have suggested that HS can occur in children as young as 6-8 years old, with a reported prevalence ranging from 0.05% to 4% in the pediatric population.

The age of onset is a crucial consideration in pediatric Hidradenitis Suppurativa, as the condition may present differently and have a unique impact on the physical, emotional, and social development of the affected child or adolescent.

Hormonal Influences and Pubertal Timing

One of the key distinguishing features of pediatric Hidradenitis Suppurativa is the potential role of hormonal factors in the development and progression of the condition. In children and adolescents, the onset and course of HS may be influenced by the timing and patterns of pubertal development, as well as any underlying hormonal imbalances or disorders.

Healthcare providers must be attuned to the potential impact of hormonal changes on the manifestation and management of Hidradenitis Suppurativa in the pediatric population, as the interplay between the condition and the individual's stage of development can be complex and require a tailored approach to care.

Unique Clinical Presentation

While the hallmark symptoms of Hidradenitis Suppurativa, such as painful lesions, abscesses, and sinus tract formation, are generally similar in children and adults, the clinical presentation of the condition in the pediatric population may exhibit some distinctive features.

For example, the localization of the lesions in children and adolescents may differ from the typical adult pattern, with a higher prevalence of involvement in areas such as the groin, buttocks, and lower extremities. Additionally, the progression and severity of the condition may vary, with some children experiencing a more rapid or aggressive course, while others may have a more indolent presentation.

These unique clinical characteristics underscore the importance of healthcare providers being well-versed in the recognition and evaluation of Hidradenitis Suppurativa in the pediatric population to ensure timely and appropriate diagnosis and management.

Specialized Diagnostic and Treatment Approaches

The diagnosis and management of Hidradenitis Suppurativa in children and adolescents require a specialized approach that takes into account the unique considerations associated with this patient population.

Diagnostic Considerations

Establishing an accurate diagnosis of Hidradenitis Suppurativa in children and adolescents can be particularly challenging, as the condition may mimic other dermatological or inflammatory conditions common in this age group, such as acne, folliculitis, or even inflammatory bowel disease.

Healthcare providers must be vigilant in their clinical examination and maintain a high index of suspicion for HS, particularly in cases where the presentation is atypical or the child or adolescent has a family history of the condition. The use of diagnostic imaging, such as ultrasound or magnetic resonance imaging (MRI), may also be helpful in confirming the presence and extent of the disease.

It is important to note that the application of established clinical staging systems, such as the Hurley Staging System, may need to be adapted or interpreted with caution in the pediatric population, as the disease course and presentation can differ from that observed in adults.

Treatment Considerations

The management of Hidradenitis Suppurativa in children and adolescents often requires a multidisciplinary approach that takes into account the unique physiological, emotional, and social needs of this patient population.

Topical and Oral Therapies

The use of topical and oral therapies, such as antibiotics, retinoids, and anti-inflammatory agents, may be the initial approach in the treatment of pediatric HS. However, healthcare providers must carefully consider the potential side effects and long-term implications of these interventions, particularly in the context of a child or adolescent's ongoing growth and development.

Biologic Therapies

The role of biologic medications, such as tumor necrosis factor-alpha (TNF-α) inhibitors or interleukin (IL) inhibitors, in the management of pediatric Hidradenitis Suppurativa is an area of ongoing research and clinical evaluation. While these targeted therapies have shown promise in the adult population, their use in children and adolescents requires careful consideration, close monitoring, and collaboration with pediatric specialists.

Surgical Interventions

In cases where conservative and medical therapies have been insufficient or the disease is particularly severe, surgical interventions, such as wide local excision or deroofing, may be considered for the management of pediatric Hidradenitis Suppurativa. However, the potential risks and long-term implications of these procedures in the developing child or adolescent must be thoroughly evaluated and discussed with the patient and their family.

Psychosocial Support and Family Involvement

Caring for children and adolescents with Hidradenitis Suppurativa extends beyond the physical management of the condition, as the emotional and social impacts of the disease can be particularly profound in this patient population.

Emotional and Psychological Challenges

The physical symptoms and visible nature of Hidradenitis Suppurativa can have a significant impact on the self-esteem, social interactions, and overall well-being of children and adolescents. The condition may lead to feelings of embarrassment, social isolation, and difficulties in maintaining peer relationships, which can further exacerbate the burden of the disease.

Moreover, the chronic and recurrent nature of HS, as well as the potential for scarring and disfigurement, can contribute to the development of mental health challenges, such as depression, anxiety, and body image issues, which can have long-lasting consequences on the child or adolescent's overall development and quality of life.

Integrating Mental Health Support

Addressing the emotional and psychological needs of children and adolescents with Hidradenitis Suppurativa is a crucial component of their comprehensive care. This may involve the incorporation of mental health professionals, such as counselors, psychologists, or child and adolescent psychiatrists, into the multidisciplinary care team.

Through individual or group therapy, cognitive-behavioral interventions, and the development of coping strategies, healthcare providers can work to support the emotional well-being of the affected child or adolescent and mitigate the potential long-term psychological impacts of the condition.

Family Involvement and Support

Given the unique challenges faced by children and adolescents with Hidradenitis Suppurativa, the involvement and support of the family are essential in ensuring the best possible outcomes. Parents, caregivers, and other family members play a vital role in:

1. Facilitating timely diagnosis and access to appropriate care
2. Promoting adherence to treatment regimens and lifestyle modifications
3. Providing emotional support and fostering a nurturing environment
4. Advocating for the child or adolescent's needs within the educational and social systems
5. Participating in the development and implementation of the overall management plan

By involving the family in the care of the child or adolescent with Hidradenitis Suppurativa, healthcare providers can empower the entire support system to actively contribute to the management of the condition and the promotion of the individual's physical, emotional, and social well-being.

Empowering Children and Adolescents with HS

In addition to the involvement of healthcare providers and family members, it is crucial to empower children and adolescents with Hidradenitis Suppurativa to take an active role in the management of their condition. This can be achieved through education, self-care strategies, and the development of self-advocacy skills.

Education and Self-care

Providing age-appropriate education to the child or adolescent with HS, as well as their family, can help to increase their understanding of the condition, its management, and the importance of adherence to the treatment plan. This knowledge can, in turn, empower the individual to actively participate in their own care, engage in appropriate self-care practices, and recognize the signs of flare-ups or complications.

Self-advocacy Skills

As children and adolescents with Hidradenitis Suppurativa navigate the educational and social systems, the development of self-advocacy skills can be crucial in ensuring their needs are met and they are provided with the necessary accommodations and support. Healthcare providers and family members can collaborate to help the affected individual learn how to effectively communicate their challenges, advocate for their rights, and seek the resources and assistance they require.

By empowering children and adolescents with Hidradenitis Suppurativa to take an active role in their care and self-advocacy, healthcare providers and families can foster a sense of control, resilience, and self-efficacy, which can have a profound impact on the individual's overall well-being and long-term outcomes.

Conclusion

Hidradenitis Suppurativa in children and adolescents presents unique challenges and considerations that require a specialized, multidisciplinary approach to care. Understanding the epidemiology, clinical presentation, and unique factors associated with pediatric HS is essential for healthcare providers to ensure timely and appropriate diagnosis, as well as the implementation of effective treatment strategies.

Beyond the physical management of the condition, the emotional and social impacts of Hidradenitis Suppurativa in the pediatric population must be addressed through the integration of mental health support and the active involvement of the family. By empowering children and adolescents with HS to take an active role in their care and self-advocacy, healthcare providers and families can work collaboratively to promote the best possible outcomes and improve the overall quality of life for this vulnerable patient population.

As we continue our exploration of Hidradenitis Suppurativa, the knowledge gained from this chapter on the unique considerations in pediatric HS will serve as a valuable foundation for understanding the management of the condition in other specialized populations, such as individuals during pregnancy, which will be the focus of the next chapter.

CHAPTER 10

H idradenitis Suppurativa and Pregnancy

Navigating the Complexities of a Chronic Skin Condition During Childbearing Years

Hidradenitis Suppurativa (HS) is a chronic, recurrent skin condition that can have a significant impact on individuals during their childbearing years. The unique hormonal, physiological, and emotional changes associated with pregnancy can influence the course of Hidradenitis Suppurativa, presenting healthcare providers and pregnant individuals with a complex set of challenges to navigate.

In this chapter, we will explore the interplay between Hidradenitis Suppurativa and pregnancy, examining the potential impact of hormonal changes on disease progression, as well as the considerations for safe and effective management during pregnancy and the postpartum period. We will also discuss the importance of preconception counseling and the development of comprehensive care plans to ensure the best possible outcomes for both the pregnant individual and the developing fetus.

By understanding the multifaceted relationship between Hidradenitis Suppurativa and pregnancy, healthcare providers and individuals with HS can work collaboratively to address the unique needs and concerns of this patient population, ultimately improving the quality of life and overall well-being of those affected.

The Impact of Pregnancy on Hidradenitis Suppurativa

Pregnancy is a time of significant hormonal, physiological, and emotional changes, all of which can have a profound impact on the course and management of Hidradenitis Suppurativa.

Hormonal Changes and Disease Progression

One of the key factors that influence the relationship between Hidradenitis Suppurativa and pregnancy is the hormonal fluctuations that occur during this time. Estrogen, progesterone, and androgen levels can all undergo dramatic changes, which may have a direct impact on the development and progression of HS.

During pregnancy, the increase in estrogen levels has been associated with an improvement or even remission of Hidradenitis Suppurativa symptoms in some individuals. This is believed to be due to the anti-inflammatory effects of estrogen and its potential to counteract the pro-inflammatory actions of androgens, which have been linked to the pathogenesis of HS.

However, the postpartum period, which is characterized by a rapid decline in estrogen levels, may trigger the reactivation or worsening of Hidradenitis Suppurativa symptoms. This "flare-up" of HS in the postpartum period is a well-recognized phenomenon and can present significant challenges for the affected individual and their healthcare providers.

Physiological Changes and Disease Management

In addition to the hormonal factors, the physiological changes associated with pregnancy can also impact the management of Hidradenitis Suppurativa. For example, the increased skin-to-skin contact and friction in areas such as the groin and intertriginous regions may exacerbate the development and progression of HS lesions.

Furthermore, the weight gain and changes in body composition that typically occur during pregnancy can contribute to the worsening of HS symptoms, as excess adipose tissue and increased friction can further aggravate the condition.

Emotional and Psychosocial Considerations

The diagnosis and management of Hidradenitis Suppurativa during pregnancy can also have significant emotional and psychosocial implications for the affected individual. The physical symptoms, potential disfigurement, and the uncertainty surrounding the course of the condition can lead to increased stress, anxiety, and concerns about the impact on the pregnancy and the developing fetus.

Healthcare providers must be attuned to the emotional and psychosocial needs of pregnant individuals with Hidradenitis Suppurativa, and integrate tailored support and resources into the overall management plan to ensure the best possible outcomes for both the individual and their family.

Preconception Counseling and Care Planning

Given the potential impact of Hidradenitis Suppurativa on pregnancy and the postpartum period, as well as the potential risks associated with certain treatments, preconception counseling and the development of a comprehensive care plan are crucial for individuals with HS who are planning a pregnancy.

Preconception Counseling

Individuals with Hidradenitis Suppurativa who are considering pregnancy should be provided with thorough preconception counseling to discuss the potential implications of the condition on their reproductive health and the management of their disease during pregnancy.

During the preconception counseling session, healthcare providers should cover the following key topics:

1. The potential impact of pregnancy on the course of Hidradenitis Suppurativa, including the likelihood of flare-ups or remission.
2. The safety and risks associated with various treatment options, including the potential impact on fertility and fetal development.
3. Strategies for managing HS symptoms and preventing complications during pregnancy and the postpartum period.
4. The importance of close monitoring and collaboration with the health-care team throughout the pregnancy.
5. The availability of support resources and the involvement of mental health professionals, if needed.

By providing comprehensive preconception counseling, healthcare providers can empower individuals with Hidradenitis Suppurativa to make informed decisions about their reproductive choices and work collaboratively to develop a personalized care plan that addresses their unique needs and concerns.

Comprehensive Care Planning

The development of a comprehensive care plan is essential for individuals with Hidradenitis Suppurativa who are planning a pregnancy or are currently pregnant. This plan should be crafted in collaboration with the affected individual, their obstetrician, dermatologist, and any other relevant healthcare providers, and should address the following key considerations:

1. Medication management: The selection and dosage of any medications, including topical, oral, or biologic therapies, must be carefully evaluated to ensure their safety and efficacy during pregnancy and breastfeeding.
2. Monitoring and surveillance: Regular monitoring of the individual's

HS symptoms, as well as the health of the developing fetus, should be incorporated into the care plan.

3. Lifestyle modifications: Strategies for managing weight, reducing friction and irritation, and maintaining proper skin hygiene should be addressed.

4. Acute management of flare-ups: Personalized plans for the recognition and management of HS flare-ups during pregnancy and the postpartum period should be developed.

5. Postpartum care: The transition into the postpartum period, including the management of potential disease reactivation and the initiation or resumption of treatment, should be carefully considered.

By working collaboratively to develop a comprehensive care plan, healthcare providers can help to ensure the safety and well-being of both the pregnant individual and the developing fetus, while also addressing the unique challenges posed by Hidradenitis Suppurativa during this critical life stage.

Managing Hidradenitis Suppurativa During Pregnancy

The management of Hidradenitis Suppurativa during pregnancy requires a delicate balance between addressing the individual's needs and concerns, while also minimizing the potential risks to the developing fetus. Healthcare providers must work closely with pregnant individuals with HS to develop personalized treatment strategies that prioritize safety and efficacy.

Topical and Oral Therapies

The use of topical and oral medications for the management of Hidradenitis Suppurativa during pregnancy must be carefully evaluated, as some treatments may be contraindicated or have potential risks to the fetus.

Topical therapies, such as antibiotics or retinoids, may be considered in some cases, as they have a lower systemic absorption and, therefore, potentially lower risk to the developing fetus. Healthcare providers must thoroughly review the available evidence and weigh the potential benefits against the risks before prescribing these treatments.

Oral therapies, such as antibiotics or hormonal medications, may be more challenging to use during pregnancy, as they have a higher likelihood of systemic exposure and potential fetal effects. In some cases, alternative treatment options, such as dietary modifications or the use of topical therapies, may be prioritized to manage HS symptoms while minimizing the risks to the pregnancy.

Biologic Therapies

The use of biologic medications, such as tumor necrosis factor-alpha (TNF-α) inhibitors or interleukin (IL) inhibitors, for the management of Hidradenitis Suppurativa during pregnancy is an area of ongoing research and clinical evaluation.

While some biologic therapies have been used off-label in pregnant individuals with HS, the long-term safety data and potential risks to the developing fetus are not yet fully established. Healthcare providers must carefully weigh the potential benefits of these interventions against the known and unknown risks, and engage in thorough discussions with the pregnant individual to arrive at the most appropriate treatment decisions.

In cases where the use of biologic therapies is deemed necessary, close monitoring of both the individual and the fetus is crucial to ensure the safety and well-being of all parties.

Surgical Interventions

The role of surgical interventions, such as wide local excision or deroofing, in the management of Hidradenitis Suppurativa during pregnancy is generally limited, as these procedures may pose increased risks to the pregnant individual and the developing fetus.

In rare cases, where conservative and medical therapies have been insufficient, and the disease is severely debilitating, healthcare providers may consider surgical options. However, the decision to pursue surgical interventions during pregnancy must be made with extreme caution and in close consultation with the affected individual, the obstetrician, and the surgical team.

Postpartum Considerations

The postpartum period is a critical time for individuals with Hidradenitis Suppurativa, as the rapid hormonal changes and physiological adjustments can lead to a reactivation or worsening of their condition.

Monitoring and Management of Flare-ups

During the postpartum period, healthcare providers should closely monitor individuals with HS for the development of flare-ups or the recurrence of symptoms. Personalized management plans, developed during the preconception and pregnancy stages, should be implemented to address any acute exacerbations and prevent the escalation of the condition.

This may involve the use of appropriate topical or oral therapies, the management of any secondary infections, and the implementation of lifestyle modifications to minimize the risk of flare-ups.

Considerations for Breastfeeding

The impact of Hidradenitis Suppurativa on breastfeeding, and the safety of various treatments during this time, must be carefully evaluated. Healthcare providers should work closely with the affected individual to assess the potential risks and benefits of continuing or resuming certain therapies, such as topical or oral medications, while the individual is breastfeeding.

In some cases, modifications to the treatment plan or the temporary discontinuation of certain medications may be necessary to ensure the safety of the breastfed infant. Regular monitoring and collaboration with a lactation specialist can help to navigate these complex decisions.

Emotional and Psychosocial Support

The postpartum period can be a particularly challenging time for individuals with Hidradenitis Suppurativa, as they may be coping with the physical and emotional changes associated with both the condition and the transition to parenthood.

Healthcare providers should be attuned to the potential mental health needs of these individuals and integrate appropriate support, such as counseling, support groups, or referrals to mental health professionals, into the overall postpartum management plan.

By addressing the physical, emotional, and psychosocial needs of individuals with Hidradenitis Suppurativa during the postpartum period, healthcare providers can help to ensure a smooth transition and promote the best possible outcomes for both the affected individual and their family.

Conclusion

Navigating the complexities of Hidradenitis Suppurativa during pregnancy and the postpartum period requires a comprehensive, multidisciplinary approach that prioritizes the safety and well-being of both the affected individual and the developing fetus.

The unique hormonal, physiological, and emotional changes associated with pregnancy can significantly impact the course of Hidradenitis Suppurativa, potentially leading to flare-ups, remissions, or other complications. Healthcare providers must work closely with pregnant individuals with HS to develop personalized care plans that address these considerations, while also minimizing the potential risks of various treatment options.

Preconception counseling and the development of comprehensive care plans are essential in empowering individuals with Hidradenitis Suppurativa to make informed decisions about their reproductive choices and manage their condition throughout the pregnancy and postpartum periods. Ongoing monitoring, the implementation of appropriate treatment strategies, and the provision of emotional and psychosocial support are crucial for ensuring the best possible outcomes for this patient population.

As we continue our exploration of Hidradenitis Suppurativa, the knowledge gained from this chapter on the unique considerations surrounding pregnancy will serve as a foundation for understanding the role of other factors, such as nutrition and complementary therapies, in the management of this chronic, debilitating skin condition.

CHAPTER 11

Nutrition and Complementary Therapies for Hidradenitis Suppurativa

Exploring the Role of Diet, Supplements, and Mind-Body Practices in Comprehensive Care

While traditional medical interventions, such as topical treatments, oral therapies, and advanced therapies, play a crucial role in the management of Hidradenitis Suppurativa (HS), the potential benefits of nutrition, supplements, and complementary therapies have gained increasing attention in recent years. These holistic approaches can serve as valuable adjuncts to conventional treatment strategies, potentially enhancing the overall well-being and quality of life for individuals living with this chronic, debilitating skin condition.

In this chapter, we will delve into the role of anti-inflammatory dietary modifications, herbal remedies and supplements, and mind-body practices in the comprehensive care of Hidradenitis Suppurativa. By understanding the potential mechanisms of action, evidence-based efficacy, and appropriate integration of these complementary approaches, healthcare providers and individuals with HS can work collaboratively to develop personalized management plans that address the diverse needs and preferences of those affected by this complex condition.

Anti-Inflammatory Dietary Modifications

The relationship between diet and the management of Hidradenitis Suppurativa has been an area of growing interest, with mounting evidence suggesting that certain dietary modifications may have a positive impact on the course of the condition.

The Underlying Rationale

Hidradenitis Suppurativa is characterized by chronic inflammation, which is believed to play a central role in the development and progression of the condition. Given that diet can influence the body's inflammatory response, the exploration of anti-inflammatory dietary approaches has become a focus in the management of HS.

The premise behind anti-inflammatory dietary modifications for Hidradenitis Suppurativa is that the incorporation of foods and nutrients with known anti-inflammatory properties may help to reduce the underlying inflammation, potentially leading to a reduction in the severity and frequency of HS symptoms.

Key Dietary Considerations

Some of the key dietary considerations in the management of Hidradenitis Suppurativa include:

1. Increased intake of anti-inflammatory foods: These may include fruits, vegetables, whole grains, fatty fish, and foods rich in omega-3 fatty acids, which have been shown to have anti-inflammatory effects.

2. Reduction of pro-inflammatory foods: Foods high in refined carbohydrates, unhealthy fats (such as trans fats and saturated fats), and certain dairy products may contribute to increased inflammation and should be limited.

3. Identification and avoidance of potential trigger foods: Some individuals

with HS may have sensitivities or intolerances to specific foods that can exacerbate their symptoms, and the identification and elimination of these triggers can be beneficial.

4. Maintenance of a healthy weight: Given the strong association between obesity and Hidradenitis Suppurativa, weight management through a balanced, anti-inflammatory diet can be an important component of comprehensive care.

Evidence and Potential Benefits

While the research on the specific dietary management of Hidradenitis Suppurativa is still evolving, several studies have suggested potential benefits of anti-inflammatory dietary approaches:

- Reduction in HS lesion counts and severity: Some studies have shown that the adoption of an anti-inflammatory diet, such as the Mediterranean diet, can lead to a decrease in the number and severity of HS lesions.

- Improved quality of life: Dietary modifications that reduce inflammation may have a positive impact on the overall well-being and quality of life for individuals living with Hidradenitis Suppurativa.

- Potential synergistic effects with conventional therapies: Combining anti-inflammatory dietary changes with traditional medical interventions may enhance the effectiveness of the overall management plan.

It is important to note that the specific dietary needs and preferences of each individual with Hidradenitis Suppurativa may vary, and healthcare providers should work closely with their patients to develop personalized nutritional strategies that address their unique circumstances and goals.

Herbal Remedies and Supplements

In addition to dietary modifications, the use of herbal remedies and dietary supplements has also been explored as a potential complement to the management of Hidradenitis Suppurativa.

Herbal Remedies

Several herbal preparations have been investigated for their potential benefits in the context of Hidradenitis Suppurativa, including:

1. Curcumin (from turmeric): This potent anti-inflammatory compound has demonstrated promising results in the management of HS symptoms.

2. Green tea extract: The polyphenols and antioxidants in green tea may have beneficial effects on the inflammatory processes underlying Hidradenitis Suppurativa.

3. Boswellia serrata: This herb, known for its anti-inflammatory properties, has been studied for its potential role in HS management.

4. Tea tree oil: The antimicrobial and anti-inflammatory qualities of tea tree oil have led to its investigation as a topical treatment for HS.

While the evidence for the efficacy of these herbal remedies in the management of Hidradenitis Suppurativa is still limited, some individuals may find them to be a helpful complement to their overall treatment plan.

Dietary Supplements

In addition to herbal remedies, various dietary supplements have also been explored for their potential benefits in the context of Hidradenitis Suppurativa, including:

1. Omega-3 fatty acids: The anti-inflammatory properties of omega-3s, such as those found in fish oil, have led to their investigation as a potential supplement for HS.

2. Zinc: This essential mineral has been studied for its potential role in wound healing and immune function, which may be relevant in the management of Hidradenitis Suppurativa.

3. Vitamin D: Low levels of vitamin D have been associated with Hidradenitis Suppurativa, and supplementation may have a positive impact on the condition.

4. Probiotics: The modulation of the gut microbiome through probiotic supplements has been explored as a potential approach to managing the inflammatory processes in HS.

As with herbal remedies, the evidence for the efficacy of dietary supplements in the management of Hidradenitis Suppurativa is still evolving, and healthcare providers should carefully evaluate the potential benefits and risks before recommending their use.

Considerations and Cautions

When incorporating herbal remedies and dietary supplements into the management of Hidradenitis Suppurativa, it is essential to consider the following:

- Potential interactions with conventional medications: Herbal and supplement use may interact with prescribed therapies, and healthcare providers should be made aware of all the products an individual is taking.

- Quality and safety: Not all herbal and supplement products are regulated, and it is crucial to source high-quality, reputable brands to ensure safety and efficacy.

- Individualized approach: The response to herbal remedies and supplements may vary among individuals, and healthcare providers should work closely with their patients to monitor the effectiveness and tolerability of these complementary therapies.

- Discontinuation of conventional treatments: Individuals should never discontinue or replace their prescribed HS treatments without first consulting their healthcare provider, as this could lead to worsening of the condition.

By approaching the use of herbal remedies and dietary supplements with caution and in close collaboration with their healthcare team, individuals with Hidradenitis Suppurativa can explore the potential benefits of these complementary approaches while ensuring their safety and overall well-being.

Mind-Body Practices and Stress Management

The chronic, recurrent nature of Hidradenitis Suppurativa and its significant impact on an individual's physical and emotional well-being have led to an increased interest in the role of mind-body practices and stress management techniques in the comprehensive care of this condition.

Stress and Hidradenitis Suppurativa

As discussed in previous chapters, chronic stress has been identified as a potential trigger or exacerbating factor for Hidradenitis Suppurativa. The relationship between stress and the condition is believed to be mediated, in part, through the impact of stress on the immune system and inflammatory pathways.

By incorporating stress management and mind-body practices into the overall management plan for individuals with HS, healthcare providers can help to address the emotional and psychological burdens of the condition, potentially mitigating the risk of flare-ups and improving the individual's overall quality of life.

Mind-Body Practices and Their Benefits

Various mind-body practices have been explored for their potential benefits in the context of Hidradenitis Suppurativa, including:

1. Mindfulness and meditation: The practice of mindfulness and meditation has been shown to have a positive impact on reducing stress, anxiety, and inflammation, which may be beneficial for individuals with HS.

2. Relaxation techniques: Methods such as deep breathing, progressive muscle relaxation, and guided imagery can help to elicit the body's relaxation response and mitigate the effects of stress.

3. Yoga and tai chi: These gentle, mind-body exercises can promote physical and mental well-being, potentially offering benefits for individuals with Hidradenitis Suppurativa.

4. Biofeedback: This technique, which involves the use of electronic devices to provide real-time feedback on physiological processes, can help individuals learn to control and manage their stress and anxiety levels.

Evidence and Potential Benefits

While the research on the specific application of mind-body practices in the management of Hidradenitis Suppurativa is still limited, studies have suggested the potential benefits of these approaches:

- Reduction in HS symptom severity: Some studies have reported a decrease in the severity of HS lesions and flare-ups in individuals who have incorporated mind-body practices into their management plan.

- Improvement in quality of life: Mind-body practices have been associated with enhanced emotional well-being, reduced stress and anxiety, and an overall improvement in the quality of life for individuals living with Hidradenitis Suppurativa.

- Potential synergistic effects with conventional therapies: The integration of mind-body practices with traditional medical interventions may enhance the overall effectiveness of the management plan for individuals with HS.

It is important to note that the specific mind-body practices and their implementation should be tailored to the individual's preferences, abilities, and the stage of their Hidradenitis Suppurativa. Healthcare providers should work closely with their patients to identify and incorporate the most appropriate mind-body techniques into the comprehensive management of this chronic skin condition.

Integrating Complementary Approaches into Comprehensive Care

The exploration of nutritional, herbal, and mind-body approaches in the management of Hidradenitis Suppurativa represents a growing area of interest and research, as individuals living with this chronic condition seek to optimize their overall well-being and quality of life.

However, it is crucial to emphasize that the use of these complementary therapies should not replace or diminish the importance of conventional medical interventions in the management of Hidradenitis Suppurativa. Rather, these approaches should be viewed as potential adjuncts to the overall management plan, integrated in a thoughtful and collaborative manner between individuals with HS and their healthcare providers.

When incorporating complementary therapies into the care of individuals with Hidradenitis Suppurativa, healthcare providers should:

1. Thoroughly evaluate the available evidence and potential benefits, as well as the risks and limitations, of each approach.
2. Engage in open discussions with their patients about their interest in and experience with complementary therapies, addressing any concerns

or questions they may have.

3. Develop personalized management plans that strategically integrate nutritional, herbal, and mind-body practices in a way that complements and enhances the effectiveness of conventional medical treatments.

4. Closely monitor the individual's response to the complementary therapies, adjusting the management plan as needed to ensure optimal outcomes and safety.

5. Encourage open communication and collaboration between the individual, the healthcare provider, and any other practitioners involved in the complementary care, to ensure a cohesive and coordinated approach.

By adopting a comprehensive, integrative approach to the management of Hidradenitis Suppurativa, healthcare providers can empower individuals living with this chronic condition to take an active role in their care, explore the potential benefits of complementary therapies, and ultimately achieve improved physical, emotional, and overall well-being.

Conclusion

The exploration of nutritional, herbal, and mind-body practices in the management of Hidradenitis Suppurativa represents a growing area of interest and research, as individuals living with this chronic, debilitating condition seek to optimize their overall well-being and quality of life.

The anti-inflammatory properties of certain dietary modifications, the potential benefits of herbal remedies and dietary supplements, and the role of mind-body practices in addressing the emotional and psychological aspects of HS have all been the subject of increasing attention and investigation.

While the evidence for the efficacy of these complementary approaches in the management of Hidradenitis Suppurativa is still evolving, the integration of these therapies into a comprehensive, personalized management plan can serve as a valuable adjunct to conventional medical interventions, potentially enhancing the overall effectiveness of the care provided to individuals living with this chronic skin condition.

Healthcare providers must approach the incorporation of complementary therapies with care, thoroughly evaluating the available evidence, addressing any concerns or questions their patients may have, and working collaboratively to develop personalized management strategies that prioritize safety, efficacy, and the individual's unique needs and preferences.

By embracing an integrative, holistic approach to the management of Hidradenitis Suppurativa, we can empower individuals affected by this condition to take an active role in their care, explore the potential benefits of complementary therapies, and ultimately achieve improved physical, emotional, and overall well-being.

CHAPTER 12

Emerging Research and Future Directions in Hidradenitis Suppurativa

Unlocking New Frontiers for Improved Patient Outcomes

The field of Hidradenitis Suppurativa (HS) research is rapidly evolving, with ongoing investigations aimed at uncovering novel treatment targets, improving diagnostic and management strategies, and enhancing the overall quality of life for those living with this chronic, debilitating skin condition. As our understanding of the underlying mechanisms and pathogenesis of Hidradenitis Suppurativa continues to expand, healthcare providers and researchers are poised to unlock new frontiers in the care and support of this patient population.

In this chapter, we will explore the latest advancements in Hidradenitis Suppurativa research, delving into the emerging therapies, diagnostic tools, and patient-centered approaches that hold promise for improving outcomes and empowering individuals affected by this condition. Additionally, we will examine the implications of these innovations and the potential impact they may have on the future of HS management.

By staying at the forefront of the evolving landscape in Hidradenitis Suppurativa research, healthcare providers and individuals living with HS can work collaboratively to capitalize on the latest developments and optimize the care and support provided to those affected by this complex skin disease.

Emerging Therapeutic Targets and Novel Treatments

One of the most exciting areas of Hidradenitis Suppurativa research is the exploration of novel therapeutic targets and the development of innovative treatment modalities. As our understanding of the underlying pathogenesis of HS continues to expand, researchers are identifying new molecular pathways and potential targets for intervention, which may lead to the emergence of more effective, targeted therapies.

Targeting Inflammatory Pathways

The central role of chronic inflammation in the development and progression of Hidradenitis Suppurativa has been a key focus of research, with ongoing investigations exploring the inhibition of specific inflammatory mediators and pathways as potential therapeutic strategies.

Beyond the currently available biologic therapies that target tumor necrosis factor-alpha (TNF-α) or interleukins (ILs), researchers are exploring the potential of targeting other inflammatory cytokines, such as IL-1, IL-6, and IL-23, as well as the inhibition of signaling pathways like the Janus kinase (JAK)/signal transducer and activator of transcription (STAT) axis.

The development of these novel, targeted anti-inflammatory therapies holds promise for improved efficacy and potentially fewer side effects compared to traditional systemic treatments, particularly for individuals with moderate to severe Hidradenitis Suppurativa.

Modulating Cellular Processes

In addition to targeting inflammatory pathways, researchers are also investigating the potential of therapies that aim to disrupt the underlying cellular processes involved in the pathogenesis of Hidradenitis Suppurativa.

For instance, the inhibition of gamma-secretase, an enzyme complex implicated in the regulation of cellular signaling and inflammation, has emerged as a promising therapeutic target for HS. By modulating the gamma-secretase pathway, researchers hope to address the fundamental drivers of the condition and potentially halt or reverse the disease progression.

Furthermore, the exploration of therapies that target the processes of follicular occlusion and hyperkeratosis, which are hallmarks of Hidradenitis Suppurativa, may lead to the development of novel treatment approaches that address the root causes of the condition.

Innovative Delivery Mechanisms

Alongside the identification of new therapeutic targets, researchers are also exploring innovative delivery mechanisms to enhance the effectiveness and patient-centered approach to Hidradenitis Suppurativa treatments.

One example is the development of sustained-release or long-acting formulations of existing therapies, such as biologics or antibiotics, which could potentially improve adherence, reduce the frequency of administration, and provide more consistent disease control for individuals with HS.

Additionally, the investigation of alternative routes of administration, such as intralesional injections or transdermal delivery systems, may offer more targeted and convenient treatment options, particularly for individuals with localized or recurrent disease manifestations.

Ongoing Clinical Trials and Promising Developments

The pursuit of these emerging therapeutic targets and innovative treatment approaches for Hidradenitis Suppurativa is evident in the growing number of ongoing clinical trials and the promising developments in the research pipeline.

Numerous clinical trials are currently evaluating the safety and efficacy of novel biologic agents, small-molecule inhibitors, and combination therapies in the management of Hidradenitis Suppurativa. These studies are exploring the potential of targeting a wide range of inflammatory pathways, cellular processes, and delivery mechanisms, with the goal of improving patient outcomes and expanding the treatment options available for this chronic, debilitating condition.

As these clinical trials progress and the results become available, healthcare providers and individuals living with Hidradenitis Suppurativa can look forward to the potential incorporation of these innovative therapies into the standard of care, offering new hope and improved disease management strategies.

Advancements in Diagnosis and Assessment

In addition to the development of novel treatment approaches, the field of Hidradenitis Suppurativa research is also witnessing advancements in diagnostic and assessment tools, which can facilitate earlier identification, more accurate staging, and personalized management of the condition.

Improved Diagnostic Techniques
   One of the key areas of research in HS diagnostics is the exploration of novel biomarkers and imaging modalities that can enhance the recognition and characterization of the condition.

For instance, the investigation of specific genetic or inflammatory markers that may be associated with Hidradenitis Suppurativa could lead to the development of diagnostic tests that improve the accuracy and timeliness of the diagnosis, potentially addressing the issue of underdiagnosis that has plagued this condition.

Additionally, the advancement of imaging techniques, such as high-resolution ultrasound or magnetic resonance imaging (MRI), may provide healthcare providers with more detailed and objective assessments of the extent and severity of HS, guiding the selection of appropriate treatment strategies and monitoring disease progression.

These diagnostic advancements hold the potential to not only improve the recognition of Hidradenitis Suppurativa but also enable more personalized and targeted approaches to the management of the condition.

Enhanced Disease Staging and Monitoring

Alongside improved diagnostic tools, researchers are also exploring the development of more comprehensive and accurate disease staging and monitoring systems for Hidradenitis Suppurativa.

While the Hurley Staging System is currently the most widely used clinical tool for categorizing the severity of HS, ongoing research is investigating the potential of incorporating additional parameters, such as objective measures of inflammation, quality of life assessments, and digital imaging, to create more robust and personalized staging and monitoring frameworks.

These advancements in disease assessment and monitoring can aid healthcare providers in making more informed decisions regarding treatment selection, tracking the effectiveness of interventions, and identifying early signs of disease progression or complications.

Ultimately, the improvements in diagnostic and assessment capabilities for Hidradenitis Suppurativa can lead to earlier recognition of the condition, more accurate staging and monitoring, and the implementation of tailored management strategies that address the unique needs and characteristics of each individual living with this chronic skin disease.

Patient-Centered Approaches and Quality of Life Considerations

As the field of Hidradenitis Suppurativa research continues to evolve, there is an increasing focus on the incorporation of patient-centered approaches and the prioritization of quality of life considerations in the management of this condition.

Empowering Individuals with HS

One of the key areas of research in this domain is the exploration of strategies to empower individuals living with Hidradenitis Suppurativa, enabling them to take a more active role in the management of their condition and their overall well-being.

This may involve the development of educational resources, self-management tools, and patient-reported outcome measures that allow individuals with HS to better recognize and communicate their symptoms, advocate for their needs, and collaborate with healthcare providers in the decision-making process.

By empowering individuals with Hidradenitis Suppurativa, researchers and healthcare providers aim to foster a sense of control, self-efficacy, and shared decision-making, ultimately leading to improved treatment adherence, better outcomes, and enhanced quality of life.

Addressing the Holistic Needs of Individuals with HS

In addition to empowering individuals with Hidradenitis Suppurativa, the research landscape is also shifting towards a more comprehensive, holistic approach to the management of this condition, addressing not only the physical manifestations but also the emotional, social, and psychosocial impacts experienced by those affected.

Investigations are exploring the integration of mental health support, social services, and community-based resources into the overall care of individuals with HS, recognizing the significant burden that this chronic condition can place on an individual's well-being and quality of life.

Furthermore, research is also examining the potential benefits of incorporating patient-reported outcome measures, such as assessments of pain, disease-related distress, and functional impairment, into the evaluation and management of Hidradenitis Suppurativa, ensuring that the unique perspectives and priorities of individuals living with the condition are given due consideration.

By adopting a more comprehensive, patient-centered approach, the research community aims to develop interventions and support systems that address the multifaceted needs of individuals with Hidradenitis Suppurativa, ultimately leading to improved overall outcomes and a better quality of life.

Implications for the Future of Hidradenitis Suppurativa Management

The advancements in Hidradenitis Suppurativa research, from the development of novel therapeutic targets to the enhancement of diagnostic and assessment capabilities, as well as the incorporation of patient-centered approaches, hold significant implications for the future management of this chronic, debilitating skin condition.

Improved Treatment Options and Personalized Care

The ongoing exploration of emerging therapies and innovative delivery mechanisms for Hidradenitis Suppurativa has the potential to expand the treatment arsenal available to healthcare providers, offering new options for individuals who have not responded adequately to existing interventions.

As these novel treatments are integrated into the standard of care, healthcare providers will be able to craft more personalized management plans, tailoring the selection and combination of therapies to the unique needs, disease characteristics, and preferences of each individual living with HS.

This personalized, precision-based approach to the management of Hidradenitis Suppurativa can lead to improved treatment outcomes, reduced side effects, and a better quality of life for those affected by the condition.

Earlier Diagnosis and Targeted Interventions

The advancements in diagnostic techniques and disease assessment tools for Hidradenitis Suppurativa can facilitate earlier recognition of the condition, enabling healthcare providers to implement targeted interventions at earlier stages of the disease.

By achieving earlier diagnosis and more accurate staging of HS, healthcare providers can potentially prevent or delay the progression of the condition, mitigate the development of complications, and improve the overall long-term outcomes for individuals living with this chronic skin disease.

Moreover, the enhanced ability to objectively monitor the course of Hidradenitis Suppurativa can aid in the evaluation of treatment effectiveness, guiding healthcare providers in making more informed decisions regarding the continuation, modification, or escalation of interventions.

Empowered and Engaged Individuals with HS

The incorporation of patient-centered approaches and the prioritization of quality of life considerations in Hidradenitis Suppurativa research have the potential to empower individuals living with the condition and foster a more collaborative partnership between patients and healthcare providers.

By equipping individuals with HS with the knowledge, tools, and resources to actively participate in their care, researchers and healthcare providers can help to cultivate a sense of control, self-efficacy, and shared decision-making, ultimately leading to improved treatment adherence, better outcomes, and a enhanced overall well-being.

Furthermore, the integration of holistic support systems, mental health resources, and community-based interventions can address the multifaceted needs of individuals with Hidradenitis Suppurativa, ensuring that their physical, emotional, and social well-being are addressed in a comprehensive manner.

Ultimately, the implications of the evolving Hidradenitis Suppurativa research landscape point towards a future where individuals affected by this chronic skin condition can access a wider range of personalized, targeted interventions, receive earlier and more accurate diagnoses, and play a more active role in the management of their disease, leading to improved long-term outcomes and a better quality of life.

Conclusion

The field of Hidradenitis Suppurativa research is rapidly advancing, with ongoing investigations aimed at unlocking new frontiers in the diagnosis, treatment, and overall management of this chronic, debilitating skin condition. From the exploration of novel therapeutic targets and innovative delivery mechanisms to the enhancement of diagnostic and assessment capabilities, as well as the incorporation of patient-centered approaches, the research community is poised to drive significant improvements in the care and support provided to individuals living with Hidradenitis Suppurativa.

As these advancements in HS research continue to unfold, healthcare providers and individuals affected by the condition can look forward to the potential integration of more effective, personalized treatment options, earlier and more accurate diagnoses, and the implementation of comprehensive, holistic management strategies that prioritize the unique needs and priorities of those living with this challenging skin disease.

By staying at the forefront of the evolving landscape in Hidradenitis Suppurativa research, healthcare providers and individuals with HS can work collaboratively to capitalize on the latest developments and optimise the care and support provided to this patient population, ultimately leading to improved long-term outcomes and a better quality of life for those affected by this chronic condition.

CHAPTER 13

Navigating the Healthcare System for Hidradenitis Suppurativa

Empowering Individuals to Access Comprehensive, Multidisciplinary Care

Hidradenitis Suppurativa (HS) is a complex, chronic skin condition that requires specialized, multidisciplinary care to manage effectively. However, the navigation of the healthcare system can pose significant challenges for individuals living with Hidradenitis Suppurativa, as they often face barriers to accessing appropriate care, securing adequate insurance coverage, and advocating for their unique needs within the medical landscape.

In this chapter, we will explore the various aspects of navigating the healthcare system for individuals with Hidradenitis Suppurativa, including strategies for accessing specialized care, considerations around insurance coverage and financial implications, and the importance of advocacy and support resources. By equipping individuals with the knowledge and tools to effectively navigate the healthcare system, we can empower them to take a more active role in their care and improve their overall outcomes and quality of life.

Accessing Specialized Care and Multidisciplinary Approach

One of the primary challenges faced by individuals with Hidradenitis

Suppurativa is securing access to specialized, multidisciplinary care. Given the complexity of the condition and the need for a comprehensive, tailored approach to management, individuals with HS often require the expertise of various healthcare professionals, including dermatologists, primary care providers, surgeons, and mental health specialists.

Identifying Specialized Providers

The first step in accessing appropriate care for Hidradenitis Suppurativa is identifying healthcare providers who have experience and expertise in managing the condition. This may involve:

1. Seeking referrals from primary care physicians to dermatologists or other specialists with a focus on HS management.
2. Researching and connecting with academic medical centers or specialized HS clinics that offer a multidisciplinary approach to care.
3. Utilizing online resources, such as patient advocacy organizations or healthcare provider directories, to identify HS-experienced specialists in the local or regional area.

It is important to note that the availability and accessibility of specialized HS providers can vary significantly based on geographic location, healthcare infrastructure, and the individual's insurance coverage.

Navigating the Referral Process

Once individuals with Hidradenitis Suppurativa have identified potential healthcare providers, they may need to navigate the referral process, which can be complex and time-consuming.

Strategies for navigating the referral process may include:
- Proactively advocating for referrals to HS-experienced specialists with primary care providers.

- Requesting copies of medical records and test results to facilitate the referral and ensure continuity of care.

- Contacting the specialist's office directly to inquire about the referral process and any necessary documentation.

- Persisting and following up on referral requests to ensure timely access to the appropriate specialists.

Establishing a Multidisciplinary Care Team

Effective management of Hidradenitis Suppurativa often requires the collaboration of a multidisciplinary care team, which may include:

- Dermatologists: Specialists in the diagnosis and treatment of skin conditions, including HS.

- Primary care providers: Responsible for overall health management and coordination of care.

- Surgeons: Involved in the surgical interventions for HS, such as excisions or deroofing procedures.

- Wound care specialists: Provide expertise in the management of HS-related skin lesions and wound care.

- Mental health professionals: Offer support for the emotional and psychological aspects of living with HS.

- Nutritionists or dietitians: Provide guidance on anti-inflammatory dietary modifications.

By establishing a multidisciplinary care team, individuals with Hidradenitis Suppurativa can ensure that their diverse needs are addressed, and their care is coordinated across different healthcare specialties.

Insurance Coverage and Financial Considerations

The financial implications of managing Hidradenitis Suppurativa can pose significant challenges for individuals, as the condition often requires extensive and ongoing medical interventions, which can be costly, particularly in the absence of adequate insurance coverage.

Understanding Insurance Coverage

Navigating the complexities of insurance coverage for Hidradenitis Suppurativa can be daunting, as policies and coverage levels can vary widely. Individuals with HS should be familiar with the following aspects of their insurance plan:

1. Covered treatments: Understand which medications, therapies, and procedures are included in the plan's coverage.
2. Out-of-pocket costs: Be aware of deductibles, copays, and coinsurance requirements for HS-related care.
3. Referral and authorization requirements: Determine if specialist referrals or prior authorizations are needed for certain treatments.
4. Limitations and exclusions: Identify any specific limitations or exclusions related to HS management within the insurance policy.

By thoroughly understanding their insurance coverage, individuals with Hidradenitis Suppurativa can better anticipate and plan for the financial aspects of their care, reducing the risk of unexpected costs or coverage gaps.

Navigating Insurance Challenges

Even with comprehensive insurance coverage, individuals with Hidradenitis Suppurativa may face challenges in obtaining approval for certain treatments or navigating the appeals process. Strategies for navigating these challenges may include:

- Communicating directly with the insurance provider to understand the rationale for coverage decisions and discuss potential alternatives.
- Advocating for the medical necessity of recommended treatments, based on evidence-based guidelines and the individual's specific circumstances.

- Engaging with healthcare providers to assist in the appeals process and provide supporting documentation.

- Exploring patient assistance programs or financial aid resources that may be available to help offset the costs of HS management.

Financial Assistance and Resource Availability

In addition to insurance coverage, individuals with Hidradenitis Suppurativa should be aware of other financial assistance and resource options that may be available to them, such as:

1. Patient assistance programs: Offered by pharmaceutical companies or charitable organizations to help individuals access necessary medications or therapies.
2. Medicaid or other state-based insurance programs: May provide coverage for individuals who meet certain income or disability criteria.
3. Nonprofit organizations and support groups: Can offer information, resources, and guidance on navigating the financial aspects of HS management.

By exploring and leveraging these various financial assistance and resource options, individuals with Hidradenitis Suppurativa can work to mitigate the financial burden associated with their condition and ensure access to the necessary care and support.

Advocacy and Support Resources

Effective management of Hidradenitis Suppurativa requires not only specialized medical care but also the ability to advocate for one's needs and access appropriate support resources. Individuals living with HS must be empowered to navigate the healthcare system and advocate for their rights and specific requirements.

Advocacy and Self-Advocacy

Advocacy is a crucial component of navigating the healthcare system for individuals with Hidradenitis Suppurativa. This may involve:

1. Educating healthcare providers about the condition and its impact on the individual's daily life.
2. Requesting accommodations in the workplace, educational settings, or social environments to address the physical and emotional challenges of HS.
3. Participating in shared decision-making with healthcare providers to ensure the individual's preferences and goals are incorporated into the management plan.
4. Engaging with policymakers, insurance providers, and healthcare organizations to advocate for improved access to HS-related care and coverage.

By developing self-advocacy skills, individuals with Hidradenitis Suppurativa can effectively communicate their needs, assert their rights, and collaborate with healthcare providers to ensure they receive the comprehensive care and support they require.

Support Resources and Networks

In addition to advocating for their own needs, individuals with Hidradenitis Suppurativa can also benefit from accessing various support resources and networks, including:

1. Patient advocacy organizations: These organizations provide educational resources, support groups, and advocacy initiatives to help individuals with HS navigate their condition and the healthcare system.
2. Online communities and forums: Virtual platforms where individuals

with HS can connect, share experiences, and offer mutual support.

3. Local support groups: In-person or virtual groups where individuals with HS can meet, share their stories, and receive peer-to-peer support.
4. Counseling and mental health services: Professionals who can provide emotional and psychological support to individuals living with the challenges of Hidradenitis Suppurativa.

By leveraging these support resources and networks, individuals with Hidradenitis Suppurativa can feel empowered, less isolated, and better equipped to manage the multifaceted aspects of their condition.

Collaboration and Integration of Support Systems

Navigating the healthcare system for Hidradenitis Suppurativa requires a collaborative effort between individuals with HS, their healthcare providers, and the various support resources and networks available to them.

Fostering Partnerships with Healthcare Providers

Individuals with Hidradenitis Suppurativa should work to establish strong partnerships with their healthcare providers, facilitating open communication, shared decision-making, and the integration of support resources into the overall management plan.

By collaborating with their healthcare team, individuals with HS can ensure that their unique needs, preferences, and challenges are recognized and addressed, leading to more personalized and effective care.

Integrating Support Resources into the Management Plan

The incorporation of support resources, such as patient advocacy organizations, online communities, and mental health services, should be an integral component of the comprehensive management plan for Hidradenitis Suppurativa.

Healthcare providers can play a crucial role in connecting individuals with HS to these valuable support systems, empowering them to access the information, resources, and peer-to-peer support they need to effectively navigate their condition and the healthcare landscape.

Continuous Evaluation and Adjustment

Navigating the healthcare system for Hidradenitis Suppurativa is an ongoing process that requires continuous evaluation and adjustment. Individuals with HS and their healthcare providers should regularly review the effectiveness of the support systems and advocacy efforts, making necessary modifications to ensure that the individual's needs are being met and their access to appropriate care is maintained.

By fostering collaborative partnerships, integrating support resources, and continuously evaluating the effectiveness of the navigation process, individuals with Hidradenitis Suppurativa can empower themselves to take a more active role in their care, overcome barriers within the healthcare system, and achieve improved outcomes and quality of life.

Conclusion

Navigating the healthcare system for Hidradenitis Suppurativa can be a complex and challenging endeavor, but it is a crucial aspect of managing this chronic, debilitating skin condition effectively. Individuals with HS must be equipped with the knowledge, resources, and advocacy skills to access specialized, multidisciplinary care, secure adequate insurance coverage, and leverage support systems that can address the diverse needs associated with this condition.

By understanding the strategies for identifying HS-experienced healthcare providers, navigating the referral process, and collaborating with a multidisciplinary care team, individuals with Hidradenitis Suppurativa can work to ensure that they receive the comprehensive, tailored care they require.

Additionally, addressing the financial implications of HS management, including navigating insurance coverage and exploring available financial assistance resources, can help to mitigate the burden and ensure access to necessary treatments and support.

Ultimately, the successful navigation of the healthcare system for Hidradenitis Suppurativa relies on the empowerment of individuals to advocate for their needs, leverage support resources and networks, and foster collaborative partnerships with their healthcare providers. By equipping individuals with the knowledge and tools to effectively navigate the healthcare landscape, we can help to improve their overall outcomes, enhance their quality of life, and ensure that they receive the comprehensive care and support they deserve.

CHAPTER 14

Living with Hidradenitis Suppurativa

Empowering Individuals to Reclaim their Lives

Hidradenitis Suppurativa (HS) is a chronic, recurrent skin condition that can have a profound and far-reaching impact on the lives of those affected. From the physical symptoms and limitations to the emotional and social challenges, living with Hidradenitis Suppurativa can be a daunting and, at times, overwhelming experience. However, with the right knowledge, tools, and support, individuals with HS can learn to not only manage their condition but also reclaim their lives and thrive despite the difficulties they face.

In this final chapter, we will explore the strategies and resources that can empower individuals living with Hidradenitis Suppurativa to take control of their health, build resilience, and find ways to live fulfilling lives. By addressing the diverse needs and challenges associated with HS, from physical self-care to mental health support and community engagement, we aim to provide a comprehensive roadmap for individuals to navigate the complexities of this chronic skin condition and achieve their personal goals and aspirations.

Coping Strategies and Emotional Well-being

Living with a chronic, debilitating condition like Hidradenitis Suppurativa can take a significant toll on an individual's emotional and psychological well-being. The constant pain, uncertainty, and social stigma associated with HS can lead to a range of mental health challenges, including depression, anxiety, and low self-esteem. Addressing these emotional needs is a crucial component of comprehensive care and empowerment for individuals with Hidradenitis Suppurativa.

Developing Effective Coping Mechanisms

Individuals with Hidradenitis Suppurativa can benefit from learning and implementing various coping strategies to manage the emotional and psychological impact of their condition. These strategies may include:

1. Mindfulness and relaxation techniques: Practices such as meditation, deep breathing, and guided imagery can help to reduce stress and improve emotional regulation.
2. Cognitive-behavioral strategies: Challenging negative thought patterns, developing healthy coping self-talk, and learning problem-solving skills can help individuals navigate the emotional challenges of HS.
3. Journaling and expressive writing: Putting thoughts and feelings into words can be a therapeutic outlet for individuals with Hidradenitis Suppurativa.
4. Engaging in enjoyable activities: Pursuing hobbies, interests, and pleasurable activities can provide a sense of normalcy and respite from the burdens of the condition.

By incorporating these coping mechanisms into their daily lives, individuals with Hidradenitis Suppurativa can learn to manage their emotional well-being, build resilience, and maintain a positive outlook, even in the face of the challenges posed by their condition.

Seeking Professional Mental Health Support

In addition to developing personal coping strategies, individuals with Hidradenitis Suppurativa should not hesitate to seek professional mental health support when needed. This may include:

1. Counseling or psychotherapy: Working with a mental health professional, such as a therapist or counselor, can help individuals process the emotional impact of HS and develop effective strategies for managing their condition.
2. Support groups: Connecting with other individuals living with Hidradenitis Suppurativa can provide a sense of community, reduce feelings of isolation, and offer peer-to-peer support.
3. Psychiatric interventions: In cases where individuals with HS are experiencing significant mental health challenges, such as clinical depression or anxiety, consultation with a psychiatrist may be necessary to explore medication or other therapeutic options.

By prioritizing their emotional well-being and seeking professional support when needed, individuals with Hidradenitis Suppurativa can build the resilience and coping skills necessary to manage the psychological impact of their condition and maintain a high quality of life.

Self-Management Techniques and Patient Empowerment

Effective self-management is a key component of living with Hidradenitis Suppurativa, as it empowers individuals to take an active role in the management of their condition and their overall well-being. By developing a comprehensive self-management plan, individuals with HS can learn to recognize and respond to their unique symptoms, implement preventive strategies, and collaborate with their healthcare providers to optimize their care.

Recognizing and Responding to Symptoms

One of the foundational elements of self-management for Hidradenitis Suppurativa is the ability to recognize and respond to the condition's symptoms. This may involve:

1. Monitoring for signs of flare-ups, such as the development of new lesions, increased pain, or changes in drainage.
2. Implementing personalized flare-up management strategies, including the use of topical or oral therapies, wound care, and pain management techniques.
3. Keeping a symptom journal or log to help identify potential triggers and patterns in the condition's progression.

By developing a keen awareness of their HS symptoms and the ability to respond effectively, individuals can take a proactive role in managing their condition and minimizing the impact of flare-ups on their daily lives.

Implementing Preventive Strategies

In addition to responding to acute symptoms, individuals with Hidradenitis Suppurativa can also engage in preventive strategies to mitigate the risk of flare-ups and disease progression. These strategies may include:

1. Maintaining a healthy lifestyle, including a balanced, anti-inflammatory diet, regular exercise, and stress management techniques.
2. Practicing proper skin and wound care, such as gentle cleansing, the use of protective clothing or devices, and regular monitoring of affected areas.
3. Avoiding potential triggers, such as friction, irritation, or exposure to known exacerbating factors.
4. Adhering to prescribed treatments and collaborating with healthcare

providers to optimize the management plan.

By taking a proactive approach to prevention, individuals with Hidradenitis Suppurativa can work to maintain disease stability, minimize the burden of their condition, and improve their overall quality of life.

Collaborating with Healthcare Providers

Effective self-management of Hidradenitis Suppurativa also requires a collaborative partnership between the individual and their healthcare providers. This may involve:

1. Actively participating in shared decision-making regarding treatment options and management strategies.
2. Communicating openly with healthcare providers about symptoms, concerns, and the impact of the condition on daily life.
3. Advocating for personalized care and the integration of the individual's preferences and goals into the management plan.
4. Seeking clarification and education from healthcare providers to enhance the individual's understanding of their condition and its management.

By fostering a collaborative relationship with their healthcare team, individuals with Hidradenitis Suppurativa can become empowered partners in their own care, leading to improved outcomes and a greater sense of control over their condition.

Building a Support Network and Community Engagement

Living with a chronic, debilitating condition like Hidradenitis Suppurativa can be an isolating experience, and the development of a strong support network and community engagement can be invaluable in helping individuals navigate the challenges they face.

Connecting with Support Groups and Resources

Individuals with Hidradenitis Suppurativa can benefit greatly from connecting with support groups, both in-person and online, where they can share experiences, receive emotional support, and learn from the insights and coping strategies of others living with the condition.

These support networks can provide a sense of community, reduce feelings of isolation, and empower individuals to advocate for their needs and access the resources they require. Additionally, many patient advocacy organizations offer educational resources, informational materials, and guidance on navigating the healthcare system and managing the various aspects of Hidradenitis Suppurativa.

By engaging with these support systems, individuals with HS can find a safe and understanding environment to share their stories, receive validation, and build resilience in the face of the challenges posed by their condition.

Advocating for Awareness and Change

Beyond personal support and community engagement, individuals with Hidradenitis Suppurativa can also play a crucial role in advocating for increased awareness, understanding, and change within the broader healthcare and social landscape.

This may involve:

1. Sharing their stories and experiences to help educate the public and healthcare providers about the realities of living with HS.
2. Participating in advocacy initiatives, such as fundraising events, lobbying efforts, or public awareness campaigns, to promote better access to care and resources for individuals with Hidradenitis Suppurativa.

3. Engaging with policymakers and healthcare organizations to advocate for improved insurance coverage, research funding, and the development of patient-centered care models.
4. Connecting with local and national patient advocacy groups to amplify their voice and contribute to the collective efforts to improve the lives of those affected by HS.

By actively engaging in advocacy and community-building efforts, individuals with Hidradenitis Suppurativa can not only empower themselves but also work towards creating a more supportive and understanding environment for all those living with this chronic, debilitating skin condition.

Embracing a Holistic Approach to Living with HS

Ultimately, the successful management and reclamation of life with Hidradenitis Suppurativa requires a comprehensive, holistic approach that addresses the diverse needs and challenges faced by those affected by this condition. By integrating the various strategies and resources discussed throughout this book, individuals with HS can work towards achieving a balanced, fulfilling, and empowered life, despite the ongoing burdens of their condition.

Physical Well-being and Self-Care

Maintaining physical well-being and practicing effective self-care strategies are fundamental to living with Hidradenitis Suppurativa. This may include:

1. Adhering to prescribed treatment regimens, including topical, oral, or advanced therapies, as recommended by healthcare providers.
2. Implementing personalized flare-up management plans and wound care protocols to address acute symptoms and prevent complications.
3. Prioritizing a healthy lifestyle, with a focus on anti-inflammatory

nutrition, regular exercise, and stress management techniques.
4. Utilizing assistive devices or adaptive strategies to mitigate the physical limitations and discomfort associated with HS.

By prioritizing their physical well-being and engaging in consistent self-care practices, individuals with Hidradenitis Suppurativa can work to maintain disease stability, minimize the impact of their condition on daily activities, and enhance their overall quality of life.

Emotional and Psychological Support

Addressing the emotional and psychological aspects of living with Hidradenitis Suppurativa is equally important in the pursuit of a fulfilling and empowered life. This may involve:

1. Incorporating effective coping mechanisms, such as mindfulness, relaxation techniques, and cognitive-behavioral strategies, to manage the mental health challenges associated with HS.
2. Seeking professional mental health support, including counseling, therapy, or psychiatric interventions, when needed.
3. Engaging with support groups and patient communities to reduce feelings of isolation and foster a sense of belonging.
4. Advocating for accommodations and understanding in educational, occupational, and social settings to address the emotional and psychosocial impacts of the condition.

By prioritizing their emotional well-being and accessing the necessary support resources, individuals with Hidradenitis Suppurativa can build resilience, maintain a positive outlook, and navigate the psychological challenges of their condition.

Social and Vocational Integration

Achieving a balanced and fulfilling life with Hidradenitis Suppurativa also requires the integration of social and vocational aspects. This may involve:

1. Developing strategies to manage the social challenges posed by HS, such as open communication, self-advocacy, and the cultivation of understanding relationships.
2. Exploring accommodations or modifications in the workplace or educational settings to ensure that the individual's needs are met and their abilities are recognized.
3. Engaging in social activities, hobbies, and pursuits that bring joy, a sense of purpose, and opportunities for personal growth.
4. Advocating for greater awareness, understanding, and inclusion of individuals with Hidradenitis Suppurativa in the broader social and professional landscape.

By embracing a holistic approach to living with Hidradenitis Suppurativa, individuals can work towards reclaiming their lives, achieving a sense of balance and fulfillment, and inspiring others who are also navigating the challenges of this chronic, debilitating skin condition.

Conclusion

Living with Hidradenitis Suppurativa is a complex and often arduous journey, but it is one that can be navigated with resilience, empowerment, and a holistic approach to well-being. Through the development of effective coping strategies, the implementation of comprehensive self-management techniques, and the cultivation of a supportive network and community, individuals with HS can work towards reclaiming their lives and thriving despite the challenges they face.

By prioritizing their physical, emotional, and social well-being, and by actively engaging in advocacy efforts to promote awareness and change, individuals with Hidradenitis Suppurativa can not only manage their condition but also find ways to live fulfilling, empowered lives. The path forward may not be easy, but with the right knowledge, tools, and support, those affected by HS can overcome the obstacles, redefine their narratives, and emerge stronger, more resilient, and better equipped to navigate the complexities of this chronic skin condition.

As we conclude this comprehensive exploration of Hidradenitis Suppurativa, it is our hope that the insights and strategies presented throughout this book have empowered individuals living with HS to take control of their health, advocate for their needs, and find the support and resources necessary to reclaim their lives and achieve their personal goals and aspirations. By embracing a holistic, patient-centered approach to living with Hidradenitis Suppurativa, we can work towards a future where those affected by this condition are not only supported but also empowered to thrive and live their best lives.

CONCLUSION

Reclaiming Life with Hidradenitis Suppurativa

Throughout the pages of this comprehensive guide, we have delved deep into the complex and often debilitating world of Hidradenitis Suppurativa (HS). From understanding the underlying causes and symptoms of this chronic skin condition to exploring the multifaceted impact it can have on an individual's physical, emotional, and social well-being, our journey has aimed to empower those living with HS to take control of their health and reclaim their lives.

Hidradenitis Suppurativa is a formidable adversary, presenting a unique set of challenges that can often feel overwhelming and isolating. However, as we have discovered, by arming ourselves with knowledge, strategies, and a supportive network, individuals with HS can navigate this condition with resilience, purpose, and a renewed sense of hope.

Unlocking the Mysteries of HS

At the heart of our exploration has been a deep dive into the defining characteristics of Hidradenitis Suppurativa. We have examined the hallmark symptoms, such as the painful lesions, abscesses, and sinus tracts, and explored the complex interplay of genetic, hormonal, and environmental factors that contribute to the development and progression of this condition.

By shedding light on the underlying mechanisms of HS, we have sought to demystify a condition that has long been shrouded in misunderstanding and underdiagnosis. This comprehensive understanding is the foundation upon which we can build more effective management strategies and empower individuals to advocate for their unique needs.

Navigating the Challenges of Living with HS

The burden of Hidradenitis Suppurativa extends far beyond the physical symptoms, as we have come to appreciate. The emotional, social, and occupational implications of this condition can be truly debilitating, leading to feelings of isolation, low self-esteem, and a profound impact on an individual's overall quality of life.

However, through our exploration of the diverse challenges faced by those living with HS, we have also uncovered the resilience, determination, and inherent strength that resides within this community. By recognizing the multifaceted nature of this condition and addressing the unique needs of individuals, we can empower them to navigate the complexities of HS and reclaim their rightful place in the world.

Embracing a Comprehensive Approach to Management

The management of Hidradenitis Suppurativa requires a multifaceted, patient-centered approach that considers the individual's unique circumstances and preferences. Throughout this book, we have delved into the various treatment modalities, from topical and oral therapies to advanced interventions and surgical options, each offering the potential to alleviate symptoms, prevent disease progression, and improve overall outcomes.

Importantly, we have also emphasized the crucial role of lifestyle modifications, such as weight management, smoking cessation, and stress reduction, in the comprehensive care of individuals with HS. By addressing the underlying factors that can contribute to the development and exacerbation of the condition, we can empower individuals to take an active role in their own health and well-being.

Moreover, we have highlighted the significance of integrating mental health support, social resources, and community engagement into the management of Hidradenitis Suppurativa. This holistic approach acknowledges the profound impact of this condition on an individual's emotional, social, and vocational functioning, and seeks to address the diverse needs of those affected.

Empowering Individuals to Reclaim their Lives

Throughout this book, our primary goal has been to empower individuals living with Hidradenitis Suppurativa to take control of their health and reclaim their lives. By providing a comprehensive understanding of the condition, equipping readers with effective management strategies, and fostering a sense of community and support, we aim to inspire and guide those affected by HS towards a future where they can thrive, despite the challenges they face.

At the core of this empowerment lies the recognition that individuals with Hidradenitis Suppurativa are not merely passive recipients of care, but rather active participants in the management of their condition. By developing self-management skills, cultivating collaborative relationships with healthcare providers, and engaging in advocacy efforts, those living with HS can become the architects of their own care, shaping the trajectory of their lives and inspiring positive change within the broader healthcare landscape.

A Future of Hope and Resilience

As we reach the conclusion of this comprehensive exploration of Hidradenitis Suppurativa, it is important to acknowledge that the journey ahead may not be an easy one. This chronic, recurrent condition presents a formidable challenge, and the road to effective management and improved quality of life can be arduous and uncertain.

However, it is precisely within this uncertainty that we find the seeds of hope and resilience. By equipping individuals with HS with the knowledge, tools, and support they need to navigate their condition, we empower them to face the challenges head-on, to advocate for their needs, and to find the inner strength to overcome the obstacles that stand in their way.

Through the stories and experiences shared within these pages, we have witnessed the remarkable resilience and determination of those living with Hidradenitis Suppurativa. We have seen individuals reclaim their lives, redefine their narratives, and inspire others who are also navigating the complexities of this condition.

It is this resilience, this unwavering spirit, that will be the guiding light for those who continue to struggle with Hidradenitis Suppurativa. By drawing strength from the experiences and insights of this community, by supporting one another, and by relentlessly pursuing better outcomes and quality of life, we can create a future where HS is no longer a source of fear and despair, but a challenge to be met with courage, compassion, and a renewed sense of purpose.

Embracing the Future with Confidence

As we look towards the future, we are filled with a sense of optimism and determination. The field of Hidradenitis Suppurativa research is rapidly evolving, with new therapies, diagnostic tools, and patient-centered approaches on the horizon. These advancements hold the promise of improved outcomes, more personalized care, and a greater understanding of this complex condition.

Moreover, the growing awareness and advocacy surrounding Hidradenitas Suppurativa are paving the way for a future where individuals affected by this condition are no longer overlooked or misunderstood. By amplifying the voices of those living with HS and collaborating with healthcare providers, policymakers, and the broader community, we can work to create a more inclusive, supportive, and empowering landscape for all those impacted by this condition.

In this future, individuals with Hidradenitis Suppurativa will not only manage their condition with confidence and resilience but will also find the space to thrive, to pursue their dreams, and to inspire others who are walking a similar path. They will be seen, heard, and respected, their unique challenges and triumphs celebrated as part of the rich tapestry of the human experience.

Conclusion

As we bring this comprehensive exploration of Hidradenitis Suppurativa to a close, we do so with a profound sense of purpose and a deep admiration for the individuals who have shared their stories and battles within these pages. Their resilience, their determination, and their unwavering spirit have inspired us, and we hope that their experiences will, in turn, empower and guide others who are facing the challenges of this chronic, debilitating skin condition.

Through the knowledge, strategies, and resources presented in this book, our aim has been to equip individuals living with Hidradenitis Suppurativa with the tools they need to take control of their health, advocate for their needs, and reclaim their lives. By addressing the physical, emotional, and social aspects of HS, we have sought to create a roadmap for a future where those affected by this condition can not only manage their symptoms but also find joy, fulfillment, and a renewed sense of purpose in their lives.

As we close this chapter and look towards the horizon, we are filled with a deep sense of hope and optimism. The future of Hidradenitis Suppurativa management is bright, with advancements in research, the growing awareness and advocacy surrounding the condition, and the unwavering resilience of those who face it head-on. Together, we can create a world where Hidradenitis Suppurativa is no longer a source of fear and despair, but a challenge to be met with courage, compassion, and a steadfast determination to live life to the fullest.

To all those who have joined us on this journey, we extend our heartfelt gratitude and a call to action. Let us continue to support one another, to share our stories, and to work collectively towards a future where Hidradenitis Suppurativa is not only managed but also conquered, allowing individuals affected by this condition to reclaim their lives and thrive in the face of adversity. Together, we can build a world where no one faces the burden of Hidradenitis Suppurativa alone.

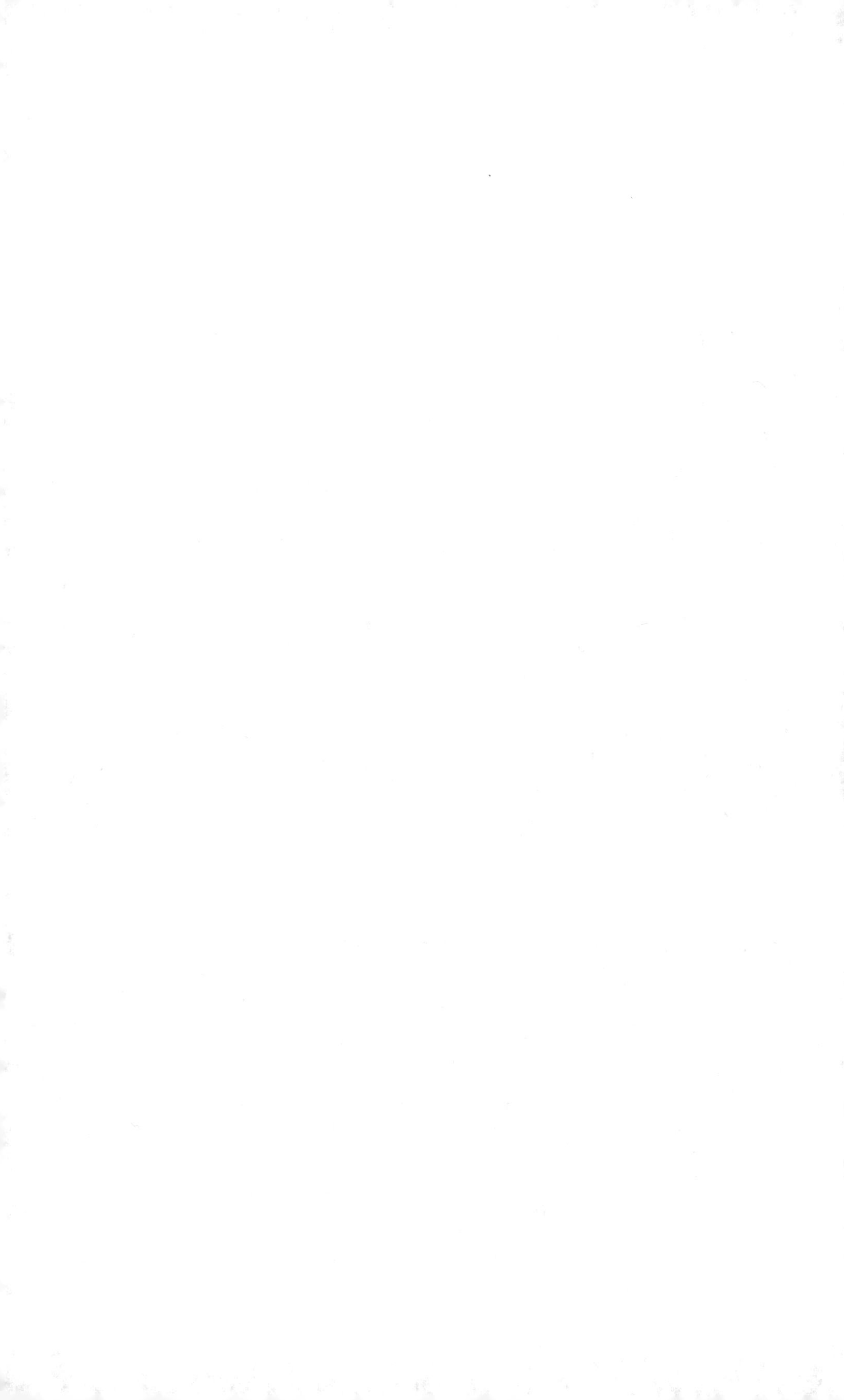

9 798334 116696